# OVID

# ARS AMATORIA

## BOOK I

EDITED WITH AN INTRODUCTION
AND COMMENTARY

BY

## A. S. HOLLIS

FELLOW OF KEBLE COLLEGE
OXFORD

OXFORD
AT THE CLARENDON PRESS
1977

*Oxford University Press, Walton Street, Oxford* OX2 6DP

OXFORD LONDON GLASGOW NEW YORK
TORONTO MELBOURNE WELLINGTON CAPE TOWN
IBADAN NAIROBI DAR ES SALAAM LUSAKA ADDIS ABABA
KUALA LUMPUR SINGAPORE JAKARTA HONG KONG TOKYO
DELHI BOMBAY CALCUTTA MADRAS KARACHI

ISBN 0 19 814441 5

© *Oxford University Press, 1977*

*Printed in Great Britain
at the University Press, Oxford
by Vivian Ridler
Printer to the University*

CONIVGI CARISSIMAE

# PREFACE

IN preparing this book I owe much to colleagues and friends. Professor E. J. Kenney allowed me to make use of his Oxford Text and also lent me an unpublished dissertation on the *Ars*. Professor R. G. M. Nisbet read the whole of the commentary, often pointing out examples of Ovidian sharpness which had escaped my notice. I remember him saying that a commentary should not be duller than the text on which it is based—an admirable objective, but hard to live up to where the *Ars Amatoria* is concerned. Dr. G. E. Rickman gave advice on historical and topographical matters, and I have profited from discussion of individual passages with Mr. M. D. Reeve. Nor does this list exhaust my obligations; some others are noted in their place. My wife typed the manuscript (latterly against the determined opposition of a small daughter), and to her, I hope appropriately, the work is dedicated.

The Introduction and Commentary were substantially completed in 1974. Therefore references to work published (or noticed by me) since then have had to be squeezed in, where possible, at the proof stage. I apologize to any scholars whose views have been treated too cursorily, or not represented at all, for this reason.

A. S. HOLLIS

*Keble College, Oxford*
*July 1976*

# CONTENTS

# LIST OF ILLUSTRATIONS

# INTRODUCTION

## *Composition of the* Ars Amatoria

THE *Ars Amatoria*, together with its companion piece *Remedia Amoris*, was the last of Ovid's love poems and indeed represented the final flowering of the brilliant but short-lived school of Roman love-elegy. Perhaps in writing it the author realized that he would be setting a seal on the whole movement; after Ovid had twisted the conventions to produce amusing but detached advice for others, neither he nor any immediately following Roman poet could well have gone back to composing 'straight' personal elegies.

To put the work in context let us retrace Ovid's poetic career up to the time of writing. He first gave public recitations of his *Amores* 'when my beard had been cut once or twice' (*Tristia* iv. 10. 58)—that is probably when he was about 18, *c.* 25 B.C. Five books of *Amores* saw the light of day, no doubt published separately. It is uncertain how long a space of time we should allow for these, but since the period included both travel abroad and Ovid's abortive steps towards a full public career, ten years do not seem too many. He followed the *Amores* with a more ambitious work, his tragedy *Medea* (now lost); *Amores* iii. 1 and iii. 15 show him feeling towards the composition of tragedy, and Quintilian's famous verdict on the play (x. 1. 98) reads like a judgement on a young writer of immense promise: 'The *Medea* of Ovid indicates to me what heights that man might have reached had he chosen to discipline his talent rather than indulge it.' But in spite of the *Medea*'s favourable reception Ovid did not turn himself into a tragic poet by abandoning lighter verse. The next decade (from about 15 B.C.) must have witnessed production of the *Heroides*, apparently not complete by *c.* 6 B.C., as well as *Medea* and perhaps other works concerning which we know little or nothing (e.g. the *Phaenomena*).

Nor had he yet finished with the *Amores*. Ovid himself felt some dissatisfaction with his earliest work (cf. *Tristia* iv. 10. 61–2 'multa quidem scripsi, sed, quae uitiosa putaui, / emendaturis ignibus ipse dedi'), and eventually he decided to publish a second edition—in three books instead of five, as the epigram standing at the front of our text informs us. The considerable reduction in size indicates that for the most part Ovid simply weeded out poems which he had come to regard as inferior. But it is probable that at least one was added for the second edition (ii. 18). There he complains that he is still not free from love-poetry; Cupid does not allow him to pursue a career as a tragedian, but confines him to lighter subjects. Several of the *Heroides* are mentioned, and also we seem to find a first reference to the *Ars Amatoria* (19–20)—perhaps so brief because the poem as yet existed only in outline:

> . . . aut *artes* teneri profitemur *Amoris*
> (ei mihi, praeceptis urgeor ipse meis).

I think 'artes . . . Amoris' should denote the *Ars Amatoria* rather than the *Amores*. These words come as close to the poem's title as dactylic verse will allow (cf. *Ars* i. 1 'artem . . . amandi'), and, although both *Amores* i. 4 and i. 8 do offer lessons in love, 'profitemur' points to a more sustained teaching role (as a description of the *Amores* it would be definitely unbalanced).[1] Whatever view is taken of this passage, one may suspect that publication of the *Amores* in a second edition moved Ovid to compose the *Ars*. His little piece on Female Cosmetics (*Medicamina Faciei Femineae*), from which only a hundred lines survive, looks like a trial run for the larger didactic poem.

Many indications show that the *Ars* was originally planned in two books, addressed to men only. To mention some of them: the table of proposed contents at i. 35–40, a pause at i. 771–2 ('half is finished, half remains'), the invocation of Erato at

---

[1] Since this statement is controversial, but the issue only marginally relevant to the *Ars*, it seems best to speak further about the chronology of Ovid's earlier works in an Appendix (I).

ii. 16 (at the beginning of the second half of the work, as in Apollonius Rhodius and Virgil's *Aeneid*), and the personal seal ending book ii as well as book iii. But after writing two books he decided to add a third for young women—by popular request, so he tells us (ii. 745–6). The *Remedia Amoris* must belong to the second stage of his conception, since it is aimed at both sexes (cf. 49–52 and numerous female *exempla*, e.g. Pasiphae, Phaedra, Scylla).

We can give more precise dates to the *Ars* and *Remedia* than to the *Amores*; *Ars* i. 171 refers to the mock sea-battle of August, 2 B.C., as having occurred 'recently', while at *Remedia* 155–6 Gaius is in the East, but seems not yet to have had his meeting with the Parthian king Phraataces which took place in the spring of A.D. 2. It is often stated that the *Ars* went through two editions, but this may be misleading. Nothing suggests that Ovid made any alteration to book i or ii (beyond adding the final couplet ii. 745–6) when deciding to write book iii and the *Remedia*. The passage on the naval spectacular and the triumph (i. 171–228) is sometimes described as written for the second edition, but for no stronger reason than that it is self-contained and can be removed painlessly; more probably the lines were composed at the last moment for the original two-book version. If indeed Ovid had made any substantial changes to the first two books, one would expect him to have obliterated signs of the two-book structure. A natural sequence is provided if we believe that he published *Ars* i–ii in the autumn of 2 B.C., went straight on to *Ars* iii with the *Remedia Amoris*, and had finished work by the spring of A.D. 2. When once Ovid had established the form and content of the poem by writing *Ars* i–ii, the addition of book iii and the *Remedia* need not have occupied him for so long.

## The Ars, Ovid's Exile, and the Poet's Intentions

Everyone knows that Ovid's exile (or more strictly relegation, since he kept his property and citizenship) was partly due to the *Ars*, and partly to a mysterious 'mistake': 'perdiderint

cum me duo crimina, carmen et error' (*Tristia* ii. 207).There-
after the poem was banned from public libraries, and it
was unwise even for private individuals to display a copy
(*Tristia* iii. 1. 59–74, *ex Ponto* i. 1. 12). For a case of relegation
the sentence was unusually severe—confinement to the remote
and insecure city of Tomis, today Constantza in Romania (I
find rather touching the piety with which modern Romanian
scholars work on Ovid). There is little point in speculating
about the 'error'.[1] The conventional choice lies between a
political or a moral offence, involving respectively Agrippa
Postumus or the emperor's granddaughter Julia. Since the
matter seems to have touched Augustus personally in some
way, Ovid refrains from speaking openly about it.[2] Even the
most popular theories run into strong and obvious objections;
without fresh evidence we can hardly hope to discover the
truth. A separate question concerns the relative weight of the
two items in the indictment. There is a tendency nowadays to
stress the *carmen* rather than the *error*, but two important
pieces of evidence point the other way. The first is a specific
statement by Ovid himself in *ex Ponto* iii. 3. 71–2, where he
makes Cupid tell him that the *Ars* contained no viciousness,
but something else (i.e. the *error*) harmed him more:

> utque haec, sic utinam defendere cetera possem;
> scis aliud quod te laeserit, esse, magis.

Then there is the puzzling gap of nearly a decade between the
publication of *Ars* i–ii in 2 B.C. and Ovid's exile in A.D. 8. The
poet alludes to this (*Tristia* ii. 545–6):

> sera redundauit ueteris uindicta libelli,
> distat et a meriti tempore poena sui.

[1] The only evidence of any value comes from Ovid himself, and this
is gathered together by J. C. Thibault, *The Mystery of Ovid's Exile*
(Berkeley, Calif., 1964).

[2] I cannot agree with Thibault (p. 20) in deducing from *Tristia* iv. 10.
99–100 that the offence was known in fairly specific terms to a wide
circle in Rome. What everyone knew was merely that Ovid had offended
the emperor (98).

During the intervening period he lived, by his own account (*Tr.* ii. 541–2), with no inkling of official displeasure. It hardly seems that the *Ars* was instantly recognized as so immoral a work that its author could not be allowed to contaminate the pure air of Italy. This sequence suggests rather that the poem was dredged up from the past at a time when Ovid faced a more serious charge, but one which the emperor found awkward to reveal. If we wonder why Ovid spent so much effort during his exile defending the *Ars*, a simple enough answer lies to hand: the *carmen* was the public and ostensible cause of banishment, and it was worth while for Ovid to justify himself in the eyes of fellow citizens. Furthermore he had a strong case in rebutting the accusation made against his poem.

The charge was quite definite: that the *Ars Amatoria* under-mined Roman marriage ('arguor obsceni doctor adulterii', *Tristia* ii. 212). I neither believe the author to have written with this purpose in mind nor Augustus really to have thought so—can he have been entirely ignorant of the conventions of love-poetry? None the less there were certain dangers in publishing a didactic poem about love under the circumstances of the time; Ovid shows himself not unaware of these, but his counter-measures proved inadequate. Throughout his rule Augustus tried to reform Roman morals by legislation; above all the *lex Iulia de Adulteriis Coercendis* of 18 B.C. made adul-tery a criminal offence with severe penalties rather than a pri-vate injury as before. The general atmosphere of the *Ars* was clearly unhelpful to this policy, and a work presented as advice to others might seem more objectionable than the straight love-elegy purporting to describe one's own experiences. In fact Ovid had provided a ground for accusation against himself whenever desired, and from exile he bewails his folly (e.g. *Tristia* ii. 316), wishing that he had burnt the poem (*Tr.* v. 12. 67–8).

He had realized the danger of being taken to recommend adultery, and sought to guard himself by means of four lines which declare that the poem has nothing to do with married women (i. 31–4). In straight Latin love-elegy (e.g. Propertius) the status of the heroine can be said to fluctuate; at one moment she resembles a Greek-style *hetaera* (a high-class courtesan perhaps of considerable artistic accomplishments), at the next a Roman lady of some social standing. This variation partly reflects the different sources from which Latin love-elegy drew, such as Greek New Comedy, Mime, and epigram. But in what seems to be definitely a Roman strand the heroine sounds like a married woman of distinction; Catullus' Lesbia may have been the prototype for such a figure, who had particular plausibility in the chaotic last few decades of the Republic.[1]

The *Ars Amatoria* is set much more sharply than the personal love-elegy of either Ovid or his predecessors Tibullus and Propertius. Accordingly it was necessary to make the young women more recognizable in a real situation too, while yet avoiding the charge of teaching adultery. So Ovid forbids married women to read the *Ars*, and indicates that the ladies he has in mind are *meretrices* (i. 435) of the class of freed-women (iii. 615 'modo quam uindicta redemit'). The government would have no interest in the conduct of these, and a long-standing Roman opinion (indeed the 'sententia dia Catonis', Horace, *Sat.* i. 2. 32) held that irregular affairs were quite acceptable provided that they did not upset marriages. In exile Ovid claims that the poem was written 'solis meretricibus' (*Tristia* ii. 303). To some extent he is made to adopt a false position there; arguing whether the work was intended *for meretrices* or *for* some other group implies that it was really meant as a serious practical treatise. But of course Ovid did not envisage that the *Ars* would be taken as a practical guide to ensnaring the opposite sex any more than Virgil expected his *Georgics* to compete with Varro's *de Re Rustica* as the standard book on agriculture. Admittedly the women in the *Ars* do not always resemble *meretrices* (take for example the 'tetrica puella' of i. 721), and we still find the 'uir' or husband[2] who

---

[1] See Gordon Williams, *Tradition and Originality in Roman Poetry* (Oxford, 1968), 528 ff.

[2] Some take the *uir* not as a husband, but as a man living in *concubinatus* with a *libertina*. That would indeed make the *Ars* more realistic

derives from the concept of the elegiac heroine as a married woman—it might have been more prudent to remove him. But these inconsistencies show not that the poet *was* surreptitiously writing for married women—rather that the work was intended in reality for no particular group, and that it drew on a full range of literary sources.

If Ovid can be acquitted on the charge of seeking to undermine sexual morality, we should by no means conclude that his poem did not intend to be provocative.[1] When he mocks recruiting difficulties in the army (i. 131–2) or advises young women to arrange their admirers in the same way as the emperor appoints to military office (iii. 525 ff.), the poet seems to be sailing close to the wind. Other respected Roman institutions also become targets for wit, e.g. the Law (i. 79 ff.), a state cult (iii. 637–8, the Bona Dea), days of national mourning (i. 413–14). But we should not exaggerate the importance of such pin-pricks and build up Ovid as a committed 'anti-Augustan' on the basis of them. The main irritation of the *Ars* to a traditionally minded Roman would surely lie in its frivolity. Romans had a strong sense of what was profitable and what a waste of time—and here is a poet presenting love as a worthy and strenuous occupation (like farming or hunting) in which all his fellow citizens should be expert!

## The Didactic Tradition

Later poets in the style, both Greek and Roman, looked back to the *Works and Days* of Hesiod as the original of this genre. Hesiod, writing in the eighth or seventh century B.C., was giving advice on agriculture, interspersed with moral maxims of a homely type. Only in the third century B.C. did the tradition really become self-conscious and assert itself; two of the best-known names are Aratus with his *Phaenomena* (on

throughout. But in the personal love-elegy the *uir* does seem to be a husband, and I prefer to view him thus in the *Ars* too.

[1] I have dealt with this and following topics more fully in *Ovid*, ed. J. W. Binns (London, 1973).

astronomy) and Nicander with the repulsive *Theriaca* and *Alexipharmaca* treating respectively venomous reptiles and antidotes to poison (in coupling *Ars Amatoria* with *Remedia Amoris* Ovid may cast a mocking glance at Nicander's pair). Favourite subjects for didactic verse included Farming, Fishing, Hunting, Fowling, Medicine, and Astronomy; it will be noted that Ovid draws constant analogies from these, so reinforcing the didactic atmosphere of his own work.

The language of a Greek didactic poem may be archaic (imitating Hesiod) and obscure even beyond the demands of technical subject-matter. Hesiod inspires digressions from the main theme which will probably be mythological in character, and perhaps also a canny and pessimistic outlook. Ovid to some extent reproduced the archaism in Latin by borrowing phrases at home in Lucretius and Virgil's *Georgics*. From the above account one could reasonably infer that the whole style and ethos of didactic poetry was quite unsuitable for a work about love—and so of course it is. Ovid gains his effect by parody and incongruity; the parallels cited in my commentary from such poets as Grattius, Manilius, and Oppian should be viewed in this light. The idea of a frivolous didactic poem was not new; Ovid himself had undertaken one in his *Medicamina Faciei Femineae* (on Female Cosmetics) and he mentions other examples at *Tristia* ii. 471 ff. Also poems giving instruction in love can be found in earlier Roman elegy (above all Tibullus i. 4, cf. Propertius iv. 5, *Amores* i. 4 and i. 8). But by writing an extended didactic poem on love, with all the proper mannerisms, Ovid achieves a hilarity never captured before. It is not merely a question of pedantry against passion; even the title of the work foretells the tension between love, usually conceived by poets as an overwhelming force which takes the individual by storm, and the precise skill implicit in 'ars'. From here comes the constant ambiguity as to whether Ovid's young men and women are really 'in love', or playing a game according to set rules. Some scholars have wondered whether we should extend the parallels with didactic literature to prose, e.g. saying that i. 41–262 (finding a girl) corresponds to *inuentio* in rhetoric (finding your subject-matter), or looking for resemblances between the *Ars Amatoria* and Cicero's *de Officiis*.[1] I feel, however, that this would labour the joke—something which Ovid never does.

## The Text[2]

### I. *The a' class*

Our manuscripts of the *Ars Amatoria* divide into two groups, of which the first (*antiquiores*, or a' group) is the more closely integrated. Members of this class (excluding Y, described separately below) are:

R  Parisinus Latinus 7311. 9th cent., written in France. 'Regius' of Heinsius.

O  Oxoniensis Bibl. Bodl. Auct. F.4.32. 9th cent., written in Wales. 'Oxoniensis' of Heinsius.[3]

$S_a$  Sangallensis 821. 11th cent. Contains only lines 1–230 of this book.

b  Bambergensis M.V.18. 10th cent. Contains only excerpts.

The postulated common ancestor (a') may in fact have been a

[1] See Aztert in the Teubner Cicero, *de Officiis*, pp. xxxii–xxxiii, and more cautiously Kenney in *Ovidiana*, ed. N. I. Herescu (Paris, 1958), p. 207 n. 2.

[2] My account of the manuscript tradition depends almost entirely on Kenney's article in *CQ* N.s. 12 (1962), 1–31. Information on Y (the Hamiltonensis) comes from Franco Munari, *Il Codice Hamilton 471 di Ovidio* (Note e Discussioni Erudite 9 (Rome, 1965)), cf. Kenney, *CR* N.s. 16 (1966), 267–71.

[3] It may be of interest that this manuscript was owned by Saint Dunstan at Glastonbury. The last leaf of *Ars* i (lines 747–72) is written in a different hand ('hand D', R. W. Hunt, *Umbrae Codicum Occidentalium* (Amsterdam, 1961) pp. vi, xii, xiv), now established to be that of Dunstan himself. Hunt (p. xiv) suggested that the saint copied from the original last leaf of the manuscript when it was becoming worn or difficult to read. But it is at least as likely that the leaf had been lost before Dunstan's time and therefore that he possessed another manuscript of the *Ars* from which to supply the lacuna—an intriguing possibility. We know that Dunstan was in the habit of comparing manuscripts when he could (I am most grateful to my Keble colleague Mr. M. B. Parkes for information here).

French minuscule manuscript written about A.D. 800 and containing all the amatory poems together with the *Heroides*. It is possible to reconstruct a stemma for the group as follows:[1]

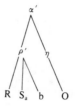

We can recover the reading of α' (i) where $ROS_a$ and b agree, (ii) where RO (one from each branch of the group) agree against $S_a$—similarly where $OS_a$ agree against R or Ob against $RS_a$. Since, however, $S_a$ does not go beyond the first 230 lines of this book, and b offers only excerpts, usually one has to rely on agreement of R and O to establish the reading of α'. In cases of conflict between R and O there has been a tendency to favour R, perhaps partly because O does not contain books ii–iii of the *Ars*, in which editors have to depend more heavily on R. But in *Ars* i there is no good reason to allow R greater weight than O (Kenney, *CQ* 1962, 15–16).

At this point one may mention the manuscript A (B.M. Add. 14086) which seems to occupy an intermediate position between the α' and β' groups, and so is regularly reported in the apparatus criticus.

## II. Y (*Cod. Berolinensis Hamiltonensis 471*) *with Selected Readings*

This manuscript cannot be called a new discovery, but it had escaped the close attention of editors through a wrong dating to the fourteenth century instead of the eleventh. The text which it offers definitely associates it with our *antiquiores* (see Munari, *Il Codice Hamilton 471 di Ovidio*, pp. 65–8). To locate it precisely in the stemma given above would not be easy; the

---

[1] The stemma is taken from Kenney (*CQ* 1962, 14). But see Goold. *Harvard Studies* 69 (1965), 7, for certain doubts.

closest links lie with R, although Y must be independent of R. Munari (pp. 20–4) gives a full collation, from which I report below just a few readings. Undoubtedly most significant for *Ars* i are the agreements with conjectures in line 133 and 558. The manuscript was used by F. W. Lenz for his Paravia 1969 and Berlin 1969 editions.

2 me        40 premenda        114 petenda        118 utque fugit uisos        126 ipse . . . timor        133 sollempni (*changed to* -nia *by either the first hand or the near-contemporary second hand*) 141 nolit (nolis *second hand*)        147 caelestibus . . . eburnis 161 tenui uento mouisse tabellam        211 quid fugis . . . uicto . . . relinques        255 bais        256 aqua (aquam *apparently second hand*)        328 uno (uni *second hand*) . . . carere (*partly in an erasure. Munari states that* placere *was the original reading, but note that* uno *fits* carere)        338 pauidi        370 ut . . . poteras 389 aut non temptasses        395–6 *omitted by the first hand* 413 tu (tum *second hand*)        439 amantum        466–71 *omitted by the first hand*        515 linguaque nec rigeat        553 steriles . . . aristas        558 reget        581 sorte tibi        592 bella        608 iuuat        620 subitur        644 magis . . . pudenda        650 adfuso 662 uda        684 duas        702 posito . . . colo        714 corrupit        715 abscedere        727 fama        730 hoc multi non ualuisse putent 731 linces . . .arion        747 iacturas (laturas *second hand*)        759 orbe        761 tenuauit (tenuabit *second hand*).

## III. *The β′ class*[1]

No stemma or neat scheme can be devised for this group (the *recentiores*), which probably represents more than one stream of tradition. That the β′ tradition is independent of α′ can be most conveniently proved for *Ars* i by the omission of lines 466–71 from ROY and their inclusion in the *recentiores*. Therefore the β′ manuscripts must, taken as a class, be given due consideration, but there is little point in trying to exalt individual members (see, however, Kenney, *CQ* 1962, 17–19), and the apparatus as a rule cites them collectively (ω = all or the

---

[1] Kenney later remarked (*The Classical Text*, Berkeley, Calif., 1974, p. 134) that these MSS. should rather be labelled 'non-α′', as it is most unlikely that all descend from a single common source.

majority, $\varsigma$ = a smaller number or a few). Only when there is nothing to choose between readings on the ground of sense may the greater over-all merit of the $\alpha'$ class be allowed to tip the balance. As with other works of Ovid, truth may lie in the most unlikely places; sometimes even a few of the *recentiores* preserve the correct reading, against both the $\alpha'$ tradition and the majority of *recentiores*. Kenney (*CQ* 1962, 19–20) provides a very useful table for *Ars* i showing how arbitrary and inconstant are the groupings of manuscripts in transmitting truth and error.

## IV. *This Edition and the Oxford Text*

I am grateful both to the Delegates of the Press and to Professor E. J. Kenney for permission to make use of the Oxford Text. This has necessitated minor adjustments to the apparatus criticus—e.g. removing references to the OCT Appendix, not reprinted here, and also some of Kenney's personal comments. Sometimes the resulting gap in the apparatus has been closed up; in other cases it has been possible to add a manuscript reading or conjecture. I much regret not having been able to incorporate the readings of Y into the apparatus criticus, but this would have added substantially to the cost and economy plays an ever increasing part in classical publishing if the price is to be remotely within the reach of students.

The opportunity has been taken, however, to make two one-letter changes which Kenney has approved since publishing his edition: 'sollemni' rather than 'sollemnia' (133) and 'reget' rather than 'reges' (558)—both of these conjectures now found to be the reading of Y. I also adopt significantly different punctuation at 80–2 and 359–60.

# SIGLA

$\omega =$ codices praeter $RrOS_aAa$ omnes uel plures
$\varsigma =$ eorundem aliquot uel pauci

### Florilegia, excerpta, fragmenta

$e =$ Escorialensis Q. I. 14, saec. xiv in.
$p_1 =$ Parisinus Latinus 7647, saec. xii ex.
$p_3 =$ Parisinus Latinus 17903, saec. xiii
$\phi =$ horum consensus

$b =$ Bambergensis M. V. 18, saec. x
$l =$ Laurentianus 66, 40, saec. ix
$o =$ Oxoniensis Bibl. Bodl. Rawl. Q. d. 19, saec. xiii
$p_2 =$ Parisinus Latinus 15155, saec. xiii
*exc. Put.* = excerpta Puteani ⎫
*exc. Scal.* = excerpta Scaligeri ⎭ ab Heinsio laudata

### Scholia

*Schol. Haun.* = commentarius in Haunensi Bibl. Reg. S. 2015
4$^{to}$ traditus, saec. xi/xii

# P. OVIDI NASONIS ARTIS AMATORIAE

## LIBER PRIMVS

Sɪ ǫvɪs in hoc artem populo non nouit amandi,
    hoc legat et lecto carmine doctus amet.
arte citae ueloque rates remoque mouentur,
    arte leues currus: arte regendus Amor.
curribus Automedon lentisque erat aptus habenis,      5
    Tiphys in Haemonia puppe magister erat:
me Venus artificem tenero praefecit Amori;
    Tiphys et Automedon dicar Amoris ego.
ille quidem ferus est et qui mihi saepe repugnet;
    sed puer est, aetas mollis et apta regi.      10
Phillyrides puerum cithara perfecit Achillem
    atque animos placida contudit arte feros.
qui totiens socios, totiens exterruit hostes,
    creditur annosum pertimuisse senem;
quas Hector sensurus erat, poscente magistro      15
    uerberibus iussas praebuit ille manus.
Aeacidae Chiron, ego sum praeceptor Amoris;
    saeuus uterque puer, natus uterque dea.
sed tamen et tauri ceruix oneratur aratro,
    frenaque magnanimi dente teruntur equi:      20
et mihi cedet Amor, quamuis mea uulneret arcu
    pectora, iactatas excutiatque faces;

ouidii nasonis artis amatoriae liber primus incipit *R* (*litt. grand.*) *O*,
ꜰᴇʟɪᴄ⟨ɪᴛᴇʀ⟩ *add. r. cf. Sen. Contr.* III vii 2, *Eutych. G.L.* vii 473.5 *K.*
2 hoc *ROS*$_a$*aHO*$_g$*l*: me *Aω*     3 mouentur *ROS*$_a$*abꜱl*: reguntur *Aωϕ*
4 leues *raꜱ*: leuis *ROS*$_a$*Abωϕl*     9 repugnet *ROA*$_a$: repugnat *S*$_a$*Aω*
11 perfecit *RS*$_a$*U*: praefecit *rOAω*     12 placida *RS*$_a$$^1$*Aω*: molli *OS*$_a$
(*u.l.*) *ꜱ*     13 exterruit *RS*$_a$*Aω*: perterruit *OS*$_a$ (*u.l.*) *ꜱ*     21 cedet
*OaA*$_a$*D*: cedit *RS*$_a$*Abω*

quo me fixit Amor, quo me uiolentius ussit,
   hoc melior facti uulneris ultor ero.
non ego, Phoebe, datas a te mihi mentiar artes,              25
   nec nos aeriae uoce monemur auis,
nec mihi sunt uisae Clio Cliusque sorores
   seruanti pecudes uallibus, Ascra, tuis;
usus opus mouet hoc: uati parete perito;
   uera canam. coeptis, mater Amoris, ades.               30
este procul, uittae tenues, insigne pudoris,
   quaeque tegis medios instita longa pedes:
nos Venerem tutam concessaque furta canemus
   inque meo nullum carmine crimen erit.

Principio, quod amare uelis, reperire labora,              35
   qui noua nunc primum miles in arma uenis;
proximus huic labor est placitam exorare puellam;
   tertius, ut longo tempore duret amor.
hic modus; haec nostro signabitur area curru;
   haec erit admissa meta premenda rota.              40

Dvm licet et loris passim potes ire solutis,
   elige cui dicas 'tu mihi sola places.'
haec tibi non tenues ueniet delapsa per auras;
   quaerenda est oculis apta puella tuis.
scit bene uenator, ceruis ubi retia tendat;             45
   scit bene, qua frendens ualle moretur aper;
aucupibus noti frutices; qui sustinet hamos,
   nouit quae multo pisce natentur aquae:
tu quoque, materiam longo qui quaeris amori,
   ante frequens quo sit disce puella loco.             50

---

24 melior $ROS_a\omega$: melius $A\varsigma$        25 mentiar $ROS_aA\varsigma$: mentior $\varsigma$
26 monemur $ROS_aA\omega$: mouemur $\varsigma$ (*sed sunt nonnulli diiudicatu difficiles*)
27 cliusque $RO$: cliosque $rS_aA\omega$        29 mouet $ROS_aA\varsigma$: monet $\varsigma$.
cf. 26        37 placitam $ROA\varsigma$: placidam $S_abs\varsigma$        40 premenda
$RS_aA\varsigma$: terenda $rO\omega$: tenenda $B^2$ (*u.l.*) $O_a$

non ego quaerentem uento dare uela iubebo,
   nec tibi ut inuenias longa terenda uia est.
Andromedan Perseus nigris portarit ab Indis,
   raptaque sit Phrygio Graia puella uiro;
tot tibi tamque dabit formosas Roma puellas,        55
   'haec habet' ut dicas 'quicquid in orbe fuit.'
Gargara quot segetes, quot habet Methymna racemos,
   aequore quot pisces, fronde teguntur aues,
quot caelum stellas, tot habet tua Roma puellas:
   mater in Aeneae constitit urbe sui.        60
seu caperis primis et adhuc crescentibus annis,
   ante oculos ueniet uera puella tuos;
siue cupis iuuenem, iuuenes tibi mille placebunt:
   cogeris uoti nescius esse tui.
seu te forte iuuat sera et sapientior aetas,        65
   hoc quoque, crede mihi, plenius agmen erit.
tu modo Pompeia lentus spatiare sub umbra,
   cum sol Herculei terga leonis adit,
aut ubi muneribus nati sua munera mater
   addidit, externo marmore diues opus;       70
nec tibi uitetur quae priscis sparsa tabellis
   porticus auctoris Liuia nomen habet,
quaque parare necem miseris patruelibus ausae
   Belides et stricto stat ferus ense pater;
nec te praetereat Veneri ploratus Adonis        75
   cultaque Iudaeo septima sacra Syro,

51 uento $ROS_a\varsigma$: uentis $A\varsigma$     53 andromedan $RO_aU$: andromedon $OP_b$ (ut uid.): andromedam $S_a\varsigma$: andromaden $a\varsigma$: andromadem $A\varsigma$     53–54 portarit … sit Naugerius: portauit … sic codd.     54 uiro $ROS_a\varsigma$: uiro est $A\varsigma$     60 in … constitit $ROS_a$: et … constat in $rA\omega$     sui $ROS_a\omega$: sua $A\varsigma$     63 cupis $ROS_aa\omega$: petis $A\varsigma$     64 cogeris Itali, $aW^2$ (ut uid.), Schol. Haun. ('quia nescies'): cogeris et RO (-es et) $S_aAb\omega$: cogêre et Heinsius     73 quaque $raB_bO_b$: quaeque $ROS_aA\omega$     74 belides et r (ut uid.) $A\varsigma$: belides (et om.) $ROS_aa\varsigma$     76 sacra $ROS_aA\omega$: festa $\varsigma$ syro O (sscr.): uiro r (ut uid.) $S_aA\omega$: deo $OP_a$: de R incert. cf. 416

nec fuge linigerae Memphitica templa iuuencae
   (multas illa facit, quod fuit ipsa Ioui);
et fora conueniunt (quis credere possit?) amori,
   flammaque in arguto saepe reperta foro            80
subdita qua Veneris facto de marmore templo
   Appias expressis aera pulsat aquis:
illo saepe loco capitur consultus Amori,
   quique aliis cauit, non cauet ipse sibi;
illo saepe loco desunt sua uerba diserto,          85
   resque nouae ueniunt, causaque agenda sua est.
hunc Venus e templis, quae sunt confinia, ridet;
   qui modo patronus, nunc cupit esse cliens.
sed tu praecipue curuis uenare theatris;
   haec loca sunt uoto fertiliora tuo.          90
illic inuenies quod ames, quod ludere possis,
   quodque semel tangas, quodque tenere uelis.
ut redit itque frequens longum formica per agmen,
   granifero solitum cum uehit ore cibum,
aut ut apes saltusque suos et olentia nactae        95
   pascua per flores et thyma summa uolant,
sic ruit ad celebres cultissima femina ludos;
   copia iudicium saepe morata meum est.
spectatum ueniunt, ueniunt spectentur ut ipsae;
   ille locus casti damna pudoris habet.        100
primus sollicitos fecisti, Romule, ludos,
   cum iuuit uiduos rapta Sabina uiros.
tunc neque marmoreo pendebant uela theatro,
   nec fuerant liquido pulpita rubra croco;

   77 linigerae $RS_aHN^2$: lanigerae $OA\omega$: niligenae $a\varsigma$     79 et $ROS_aA\varsigma$:
ad $\varsigma$    possit $ROS_a\varsigma$: posset $A\varsigma$     80 foro $ROS_a\varsigma$: foro est $\omega$: (argu-
tis . . .) foris $AW$     81 qua *Naugerius*: quo $U$: quae $ROS_aA\omega$
83 amori $ROS_a$: amore $rA\varsigma$: amoris $\varsigma$     92 quodque tenere $RO$
(-que *om.*) $S_a\omega$: quod retinere $A\varsigma$     94 solitum $A\omega\phi$: solidum
$ROS_aP_a$     97 ad *codd.*: in *ed. Bon.* 1471, *edd.*

illic quas tulerant nemorosa Palatia frondes 105
  simpliciter positae scena sine arte fuit;
in gradibus sedit populus de caespite factis,
  qualibet hirsutas fronde tegente comas.
respiciunt oculisque notant sibi quisque puellam
  quam uelit, et tacito pectore multa mouent; 110
dumque rudem praebente modum tibicine Tusco
  ludius aequatam ter pede pulsat humum,
in medio plausu (plausus tunc arte carebant)
  rex populo praedae signa †petenda† dedit.
protinus exiliunt animum clamore fatentes 115
  uirginibus cupidas iniciuntque manus;
ut fugiunt aquilas, timidissima turba, columbae
  utque fugit uisos agna nouella lupos,
sic illae timuere uiros sine lege ruentes;
  constitit in nulla qui fuit ante color. 120
nam timor unus erat, facies non una timoris:
  pars laniat crines, pars sine mente sedet;
altera maesta silet, frustra uocat altera matrem;
  haec queritur, stupet haec; haec manet, illa fugit.
ducuntur raptae, genialis praeda, puellae, 125
  et potuit multas ipse decere timor.
si qua repugnarat nimium comitemque negarat,

106 positae *rAω*: posita *ROS_aς*       109 notant *RS_aAς*: notat *Oω*
110 mouent *ROS_aAω*: mouet *ς*       112 ludius *R* (ludis, *ut uid.*) *Aς*:
lydius *ς*: lidius *rOS_aaω*       113 carebant *ROS_aF*: carebat *Aω*
114 petenda *ROS_aAω* ('.*i. signa prede petende*' *Schol. Haun.*): petita *Bent-
leius, Madvig*: notamque *o*[1]       118 utque fugit uisos *rAω*: ut fugit
uisos *RO*: ut fugit et uisos *S_aDU*: ut fugit inuisos *ς*       119 lege
*ROS_aAω*: more *Burmannus ex cod. Schefferi*, *O_g*       ruentes *RS_aAω*:
furentes *OO_g*       126 ipse *ROS_aω*: ille *rAς*       timor *RS_a* (*sed u.
Comment.*) a*ÑU*: pudor *OAω*: color *F*: rubor *T*: decor *B_b*       127 re-
pugnarat *ROS_a* (*ex corr.*) *Aς*: repugnaret *B_bU*: repugnabat *S_a* (*ante corr.*) *ς*:
repugnauit *L*       negarat *Aς*: negaret *B_b*: negare *U*: negabat *RS_aω*:
repugnat *O*

sublatam cupido uir tulit ipse sinu
atque ita 'quid teneros lacrimis corrumpis ocellos?
   quod matri pater est, hoc tibi' dixit 'ero.'        130
Romule, militibus scisti dare commoda solus:
   haec mihi si dederis commoda, miles ero.
scilicet ex illo sollemni more theatra
   nunc quoque formosis insidiosa manent.
nec te nobilium fugiat certamen equorum:        135
   multa capax populi commoda Circus habet.
nil opus est digitis per quos arcana loquaris,
   nec tibi per nutus accipienda nota est;
proximus a domina nullo prohibente sedeto;
   iunge tuum lateri qua potes usque latus.        140
et bene, quod cogit, si nolis, linea iungi,
   quod tibi tangenda est lege puella loci.
hic tibi quaeratur socii sermonis origo,
   et moueant primos publica uerba sonos:
cuius equi ueniant facito studiose requiras,       145
   nec mora, quisquis erit cui fauet illa, faue.
at cum pompa frequens caelestibus ibit eburnis,
   tu Veneri dominae plaude fauente manu;
utque fit, in gremium puluis si forte puellae
   deciderit, digitis excutiendus erit;        150
etsi nullus erit puluis, tamen excute nullum:
   quaelibet officio causa sit apta tuo;
pallia si terra nimium demissa iacebunt,

---

133 sollemni *codex Berolinensis Hamiltonensis 471* (*Y*), *Madvig ex coni.*,
*prob. Kenney, Goold*: sollemnia $ROS_aA\omega$       139 a domina $ROS_abs$: ad
dominam $A\omega$      140 qua $ROS_aAbs$: quo $F$ (*ut uid.*) $U$: quam
$s$      141 nolis $RS_aA\omega$: nolit $Os$      142 quod $RO^2S_aA_bW$
(*ut uid.*): qua $A\omega$: quid $O^1$      143 hic $ROS_aA\omega$: hinc $bP_c^2$ (*marg.*):
tunc $P_c^1$      147 caelestibus ... eburnis $R$ (*ut uid.*) $OS_as$: certantibus
(plaudentibus $L^1Q^1o$) ... ephebis $rA\omega$      153 terra $ROS_aAFO_g$:
terrae $\omega$      demissa $S_aA\omega$: dimissa $ROs$

  collige et inmunda sedulus effer humo:
protinus, officii pretium, patiente puella            155
  contingent oculis crura uidenda tuis.
respice praeterea, post uos quicumque sedebit,
  ne premat opposito mollia terga genu.
parua leuis capiunt animos: fuit utile multis
  puluinum facili composuisse manu;             160
profuit et tenui uentos mouisse tabella
  et caua sub tenerum scamna dedisse pedem.
hos aditus Circusque nouo praebebit amori
  sparsaque sollicito tristis harena foro.
illa saepe puer Veneris pugnauit harena        165
  et, qui spectauit uulnera, uulnus habet:
dum loquitur tangitque manum poscitque libellum
  et quaerit posito pignore, uincat uter,
saucius ingemuit telumque uolatile sensit
  et pars spectati muneris ipse fuit.            170
quid, modo cum belli naualis imagine Caesar
  Persidas induxit Cecropiasque rates?
nempe ab utroque mari iuuenes, ab utroque puellae
  uenere, atque ingens orbis in Vrbe fuit.
quis non inuenit turba, quod amaret, in illa?      175
  eheu, quam multos aduena torsit amor!
ecce, parat Caesar, domito quod defuit orbi,
  addere: nunc, Oriens ultime, noster eris.
Parthe, dabis poenas; Crassi gaudete sepulti
  signaque barbaricas non bene passa manus.      180

---

159 capiunt animos $ROS_a\omega\phi$: a. c. $A\varsigma$       160 puluinum $ROS_aA$
b (-illum) $L^1$: puluinar $\omega$      composuisse $ROS_aA\varsigma$: supposuisse $\varsigma$
161 tenui *codd.*: tenuis *ed. Bon.* 1471      uentos $rA\omega$: uento $ROS_aO_a{}^1$
(*ut uid.*) $O_g$: uentum $T$     tabella $A$: tabellam $ROS_a$: tabellas $O_g$: flabello
$a\omega$. cf. *Am.* III ii 37–38      170 muneris $ROS_a$: uulneris $A\omega$      172 ce-
cropiasque $RS_aA\varsigma$: cecropidasque $O$ (-etasque) $\varsigma$      176 eheu $S_aA\varsigma$:
heu $RODO_a$: heu heu $\omega$: heu mihi $\varsigma$: hei mihi $E_a$

ultor adest primisque ducem profitetur in annis
    bellaque non puero tractat agenda puer.
parcite natales timidi numerare deorum:
    Caesaribus uirtus contigit ante diem.
ingenium caeleste suis uelocius annis                                    185
    surgit et ignauae fert male damna morae:
paruus erat manibusque duos Tirynthius angues
    pressit et in cunis iam Ioue dignus erat;
nunc quoque qui puer es, quantus tum, Bacche, fuisti,
    cum timuit thyrsos India uicta tuos?                             190
auspiciis annisque patris, puer, arma mouebis
    et uinces annis auspiciisque patris.
tale rudimentum tanto sub nomine debes,
    nunc iuuenum princeps, deinde future senum;
cum tibi sint fratres, fratres ulciscere laesos,                          195
    cumque pater tibi sit, iura tuere patris.
induit arma tibi genitor patriaeque tuusque;
    hostis ab inuito regna parente rapit.
tu pia tela feres, sceleratas ille sagittas;
    stabit pro signis iusque piumque tuis.                           200
uincuntur causa Parthi, uincantur et armis:
    Eoas Latio dux meus addat opes.
Marsque pater Caesarque pater, date numen eunti:
    nam deus e uobis alter es, alter eris.
auguror en, uinces, uotiuaque carmina reddam                             205
    et magno nobis ore sonandus eris:
consistes aciemque meis hortabere uerbis
    (o desint animis ne mea uerba tuis!);
tergaque Parthorum Romanaque pectora dicam

   189 tum *r* (*ut uid.*) $OS_a$: tu *R*ϛ: tunc *a*ϛ: *om. A*        191 annisque
$ROS_aO_qU$: animisque *A*ωφ      192 annis $ROS_a$ϛ: animis *A*ωφ
198 rapit *rOA*ω: parit $RS_a$: capit ϛ: tulit ϛ: petit *D*     204 alter es
alter eris $ROS_aA$ϛ: alter et alter erit ϛ: unus et alter erit *LP*ƒ

telaque, ab auerso quae iacit hostis equo.                    210
qui fugis ut uincas, quid uicto, Parthe, relinques?
    Parthe, malum iam nunc Mars tuus omen habet.
ergo erit illa dies, qua tu, pulcherrime rerum,
    quattuor in niueis aureus ibis equis;
ibunt ante duces onerati colla catenis,                       215
    ne possint tuti, qua prius, esse fuga.
spectabunt laeti iuuenes mixtaeque puellae,
    diffundetque animos omnibus ista dies;
atque aliqua ex illis cum regum nomina quaeret,
    quae loca, qui montes quaeue ferantur aquae,              220
omnia responde, nec tantum si qua rogabit;
    et quae nescieris, ut bene nota refer:
hic est Euphrates, praecinctus harundine frontem;
    cui coma dependet caerula, Tigris erit;
hos facito Armenios, haec est Danaeia Persis;                225
    urbs in Achaemeniis uallibus ista fuit;
ille uel ille duces, et erunt quae nomina dicas,
    si poteris, uere, si minus, apta tamen.
dant etiam positis aditum conuiuia mensis;
    est aliquid praeter uina, quod inde petas.               230
saepe illic positi teneris adducta lacertis
    purpureus Bacchi cornua pressit Amor,
uinaque cum bibulas sparsere Cupidinis alas,
    permanet et capto stat grauis ille loco.
ille quidem pennas uelociter excutit udas,                    235
    sed tamen et spargi pectus Amore nocet.

---

210 auerso ς: aduerso $ROS_aA\omega$          211 qui *Heinsius*: quid *codd.*
uicto $ROS_aA$ς: uictos *ra*ω     relinques $OS_aO_g$: relinquis $RA\omega$     218 ista
$ROS_aA$ς: illa $S_a$ (*sscr.*) ς          222 et $ROS_a$ς: sed *Ab*ς     225 facito
*Heinsius*: facit *R* (*ut uid.*) $OS_aO_a^1$ (*ut uid.*): facis *rA* (*ut uid.*): fac *a*ω
Danaeia *Itali*: daneia *codd.*     *post* 230 *desinit* $S_a$     231 positi $rO_a^1$
(*ut uid.*): positis $ROA\omega$: poti *Lachmann*          234 capto *Itali*: coepto
$RP_c$: cepto $OA\omega$     236 Amore, *non* amore, *edendum*

uina parant animos faciuntque caloribus aptos;
   cura fugit multo diluiturque mero.
tunc ueniunt risus, tum pauper cornua sumit,
   tum dolor et curae rugaque frontis abit.                    240
tunc aperit mentes aeuo rarissima nostro
   simplicitas, artes excutiente deo.
illic saepe animos iuuenum rapuere puellae,
   et Venus in uinis ignis in igne fuit.
hic tu fallaci nimium ne crede lucernae:                         245
   iudicio formae noxque merumque nocent.
luce deas caeloque Paris spectauit aperto,
   cum dixit Veneri 'uincis utramque, Venus.'
nocte latent mendae uitioque ignoscitur omni,
   horaque formosam quamlibet illa facit.                      250
consule de gemmis, de tincta murice lana,
   consule de facie corporibusque diem.
quid tibi femineos coetus uenatibus aptos
   enumerem? numero cedet harena meo.
quid referam Baias praetextaque litora Bais                      255
   et quae de calido sulphure fumat aqua?
hinc aliquis uulnus referens in pectore dixit
   'non haec, ut fama est, unda salubris erat.'
ecce, suburbanae templum nemorale Dianae
   partaque per gladios regna nocente manu;                    260
illa, quod est uirgo, quod tela Cupidinis odit,
   multa dedit populo uulnera, multa dabit.


HACTENVS, unde legas quod ames, ubi retia ponas,
   praecipit imparibus uecta Thalea rotis.

   244 uinis *RAω*: uino *aς*: uenis *ς*: ueneri *O*: uenere *W*     252 diem
*ω*: die *ROAς*    255 bais *O*: uelis *r (ut uid.) Aω*: de *R* incert.    256 fumat
*ROς*: manat *Aς*   aqua *Rς*: aquam *OAω*    263 ponas (-es *OB*[1]) *ROAς*:
tendas *ς*    264 thalea *RO*, cf. Seru. ad Buc. vi 2: thalia *rAω*   rotis
*R (u.l.; non r, ut uid.) Oaς*: modis *RAς*

nunc tibi quae placuit, quas sit capienda per artes,     265
    dicere praecipuae molior artis opus.
quisquis ubique, uiri, dociles aduertite mentes
    pollicitisque fauens uulgus adeste meis.
prima tuae menti ueniat fiducia, cunctas
    posse capi: capies, tu modo tende plagas.     270
uere prius uolucres taceant, aestate cicadae,
    Maenalius lepori det sua terga canis,
femina quam iuueni blande temptata repugnet;
    haec quoque, quam poteris credere nolle, uolet.
utque uiro furtiua Venus, sic grata puellae;     275
    uir male dissimulat, tectius illa cupit.
conueniat maribus ne quam nos ante rogemus,
    femina iam partes uicta rogantis aget.
mollibus in pratis admugit femina tauro,
    femina cornipedi semper adhinnit equo:     280
parcior in nobis nec tam furiosa libido;
    legitimum finem flamma uirilis habet.
Byblida quid referam, uetito quae fratris amore
    arsit et est laqueo fortiter ulta nefas?
Myrrha patrem, sed non qua filia debet, amauit,     285
    et nunc obducto cortice pressa latet;
illius lacrimis, quas arbore fundit odora,
    unguimur, et dominae nomina gutta tenet.
forte sub umbrosis nemorosae uallibus Idae
    candidus, armenti gloria, taurus erat     290
signatus tenui media inter cornua nigro;
    una fuit labes, cetera lactis erant.

268 adeste $AO_a{}^1P_c$: adesse $RO$: adesto $a\omega$     269 cunctas $A\omega$: formae $ROb$: ferme *Housman*, forma *Heinsius, perperam uterque*     278 aget $A\omega$: agat $RH^2P_a$: (blanda rogansque) cogat $O$     281 libido $RA$: libido est $O\omega$     285 qua $RO$: quo $A\omega$: ut $Q$     287 lacrimis $RA\omega$: e lacrimis $OB$: et lacrimis $\varsigma$     arbore $RO\varsigma$: arbor $A\omega$

illum Cnosiadesque Cydoneaeque iuuencae
  optarunt tergo sustinuisse suo.
Pasiphae fieri gaudebat adultera tauri;                 295
  inuida formosas oderat illa boues.
nota cano; non hoc, centum quae sustinet urbes,
  quamuis sit mendax, Creta negare potest.
ipsa nouas frondes et prata tenerrima tauro
  fertur inadsueta subsecuisse manu;               300
it comes armentis, nec ituram cura moratur
  coniugis, et Minos a boue uictus erat.
quo tibi, Pasiphae, pretiosas sumere uestes?
  ille tuus nullas sentit adulter opes.
quid tibi cum speculo montana armenta petenti?      305
  quid totiens positas fingis inepta comas?
crede tamen speculo, quod te negat esse iuuencam:
  quam cuperes fronti cornua nata tuae!
siue placet Minos, nullus quaeratur adulter;
  siue uirum mauis fallere, falle uiro.               310
in nemus et saltus thalamo regina relicto
  fertur, ut Aonio concita Baccha deo.
a, quotiens uaccam uultu spectauit iniquo
  et dixit 'domino cur placet ista meo?
aspice ut ante ipsum teneris exultet in herbis;      315
  nec dubito quin se stulta decere putet'!
dixit et ingenti iamdudum de grege duci
  iussit et inmeritam sub iuga curua trahi,
aut cadere ante aras commentaque sacra coegit
  et tenuit laeta paelicis exta manu;             320

293 Cnossiadesque *Naugerius*: gnosiades *codd.*     cydoneaeque (*uel sim.*) *ROAϛ*: sidoniaeque (*uel sim.*) ω     297 hoc *ROAϛ*: haec ϛ     301 it ω: et *RO*: fit *AFO*$_a^2$     armentis *ROAϛ*: armenti ϛ     303 quo *Heinsius*: quod *R*: quid *OA*ω. *cf. Am.* III viii 47     315 exultet *ROAϛ*: exultat ϛ

paelicibus quotiens placauit numina caesis
  atque ait exta tenens 'ite, placete meo'
et modo se Europen fieri, modo postulat Ion,
  altera quod bos est, altera uecta boue!
hanc tamen impleuit uacca deceptus acerna      325
  dux gregis, et partu proditus auctor erat.
Cressa Thyesteo si se abstinuisset amore
  (et quantum est uno posse carere uiro!),
non medium rupisset iter curruque retorto
  Auroram uersis Phoebus adisset equis.      330
filia purpureos Niso furata capillos
  pube premit rabidos inguinibusque canes.
qui Martem terra, Neptunum effugit in undis,
  coniugis Atrides uictima dira fuit.
cùi non defleta est Ephyraeae flamma Creusae      335
  et nece natorum sanguinolenta parens?
fleuit Amyntorides per inania lumina Phoenix;
  Hippolytum rabidi diripuistis equi.
quid fodis inmeritis, Phineu, sua lumina natis?
  poena reuersura est in caput ista tuum.      340

321–2 *suspicionem nonnullis iniuria mouerunt*      323 europen *ROA*ς:
europem ς: europam ς      Ion *Ehwald*: io *codd. cf. Am.* II ii 45, xix 29,
*Her.* vi 65      326 partu *O*ω: partus *RA*      328 *om.* $p_3$      et quan-
tum *ROAU*: o (ho) q. ς: a (ha) q. ς: heu q. $B_bO_g$ (*u.l.*): nam q. $O_g{}^1$: et
satis est $ep_1$    uno *rO*: unum *R*: uni $A\omega ep_1$      carere *O*: placere $RA\omega ep_1$.
*uersum esse ironice intellegendum monuit R. Pichon:* quantum, *i.e. quantulum*
329 curruque *ROA*ω: cursuque *L. Müller, LQ*      331 niso $ROA_bD$:
nisi *a*ω: *om. A*      *post* 331 *uersus aliquot spurios habent omnes quos noui*
*codices praeter* $ROO_g$: 331 *a–b* hunc (nunc *AFH*) hostem patitur cum
reliquis auibus / altera scilla maris (nouum *r*) monstrum (circes *r* (sc-)
*N*) medicamine circes (monstrum *rN*) *rA*ω; *c–d* puppe cadens (sedens
*D*) nauis facta refertur auis / succuba scilla patri recipit dum (cum
*H*) debita matri (-is *H*) a (*marg.*) *D* (*qui tamen c, b tantum habet*) *H* (*qui*
*uersus hoc ordine habet: c–d, a–b*). *ceteras uersuum formas quae in codd. recc.*
*et edd. uett. occurrunt praetermitto*      332 rabidos *RODH*[1]: rapidos
*A*ω: medios *o*      338 rabidi *RO*: rapidi *A*ω: pauidi $P_bW$[1], *edd. post*
*Heinsium, ex Rem.* 744

omnia feminea sunt ista libidine mota;
    acrior est nostra plusque furoris habet.
ergo age, ne dubita cunctas sperare puellas:
    uix erit e multis, quae neget, una, tibi.
quae dant, quaeque negant, gaudent tamen esse rogatae: 345
    ut iam fallaris, tuta repulsa tua est.
sed cur fallaris, cum sit noua grata uoluptas
    et capiant animos plus aliena suis?
fertilior seges est alienis semper in agris
    uicinumque pecus grandius uber habet.               350
sed prius ancillam captandae nosse puellae
    cura sit: accessus molliet illa tuos.
proxima consiliis dominae sit ut illa, uideto,
    neue parum tacitis conscia fida iocis.
hanc tu pollicitis, hanc tu corrumpe rogando:         355
    quod petis, ex facili, si uolet illa, feres.
illa leget tempus (medici quoque tempora seruant)
    quo facilis dominae mens sit et apta capi;
mens erit apta capi tum cum laetissima rerum,
    ut seges in pingui luxuriabit humo.                360
pectora, dum gaudent nec sunt adstricta dolore,
    ipsa patent; blanda tum subit arte Venus.
tum, cum tristis erat, defensa est Ilios armis;
    militibus grauidum laeta recepit equum.
tum quoque temptanda est, cum paelice laesa dolebit;   365
    tum facies opera, ne sit inulta, tua.
hanc matutinos pectens ancilla capillos

341 libidine *RAω*: cupidine *O*      mota *Raω*: nota *ϛ*: plena *OA*
343 sperare *RObDQ*: superare *Aω*      348 suis *ROAωφ*: suos *ϛ*
351 captandae *Itali*: captando *U*:    captatae *ROaω*: *de A incert.*
352 molliet *RAω*: molliat *Oϛ*        353 ut *RAω*: et *O_g*: an *OP_a*
360 luxuriabit *ωφ*: luxuriauit *ROA*ϛ      361 adstricta *ROaϛ*: attrita
*Aϛφ*    363 *om. A, add. a in marg.*    ilios *ROaϛ*: ilion *ϛφ*     366 tum
*rϛ*: tu *ROϛ*: tunc *Aω*

incitet et uelo remigis addat opem,
et secum tenui suspirans murmure dicat
   'at, puto, non poteras ipsa referre uicem.'      370
tum de te narret, tum persuadentia uerba
   addat, et insano iuret amore mori.
sed propera, ne uela cadant auraeque residant:
   ut fragilis glacies, interit ira mora.
quaeris an hanc ipsam prosit uiolare ministram?     375
   talibus admissis alea grandis inest.
haec a concubitu fit sedula, tardior illa;
   haec dominae munus te parat, illa sibi.
casus in euentu est: licet hic indulgeat ausis,
   consilium tamen est abstinuisse meum.     380
non ego per praeceps et acuta cacumina uadam,
   nec iuuenum quisquam me duce captus erit.
si tamen illa tibi, dum dat recipitque tabellas,
   corpore, non tantum sedulitate, placet,
fac domina potiare prius, comes illa sequatur:     385
   non tibi ab ancilla est incipienda Venus.
hoc unum moneo, si quid modo creditur arti
   nec mea dicta rapax per mare uentus agit:
aut †non temptasses† aut perfice: tollitur index,
   cum semel in partem criminis ipsa uenit.     390
non auis utiliter uiscatis effugit alis,
   non bene de laxis cassibus exit aper.
saucius arrepto piscis teneatur ab hamo:

---

370 at *Burmannus*: ut *codd.*    poteras *R*: poteris *OAω*    373 aurae-
que *Heinsius ex uno Palatino*, $O_a{}^2$: areque $O_a{}^1$: iureque *R*: iraeque *rOAω*:
Eurique *Housman dubitanter*    377 a concubitu *ROU*: ad concubitum
*rAω*    378 te parat *ROAϛ*: temperat *rϛ*    388 nec *ROAω*: ne *ϛ*
agit *ROaO$_a$O$_b$*: agat *Aω*    389 aut non temptasses *ROAϛ*: aut num-
quam temptes *r* (nonquam) *ϛ*: aut si quam temptes $A_b$: aut non hanc
temptes *N*: aut non temptabis $DW^1p_2$: ac ubi temptaris $P_b$: aut non
temptaris *Heinsius* (tentares '*Oxoniensis*'), *B* (aud)    392 laxis *ROAϛ*:
lapsis *ϛφ*    393 teneatur *ROAϛ*: retinetur *rϛ*: tenetur *a* (*ut uid.*) *B*

perprime temptatam nec nisi uictor abi.                          394
sed bene celetur: bene si celabitur index,                       397
   notitiae suberit semper amica tuae.
tempora qui solis operosa colentibus arua,
   fallitur, et nautis aspicienda putat.                      400
nec semper credenda Ceres fallacibus aruis
   nec semper uiridi concaua puppis aquae,
nec teneras semper tutum captare puellas:
   saepe dato melius tempore fiet idem.
siue dies suberit natalis siue Kalendae,                          405
   quas Venerem Marti continuasse iuuat,
siue erit ornatus non, ut fuit ante, sigillis,
   sed regum positas Circus habebit opes,
differ opus: tunc tristis hiems, tunc Pliades instant,
   tunc tener aequorea mergitur Haedus aqua;                 410
tunc bene desinitur; tunc si quis creditur alto,
   uix tenuit lacerae naufraga membra ratis.
tum licet incipias, qua flebilis Allia luce
   uulneribus Latiis sanguinolenta fuit,
quaque die redeunt rebus minus apta gerendis                     415
   culta Palaestino septima festa Syro.
magna superstitio tibi sit natalis amicae,
   quaque aliquid dandum est, illa sit atra dies.
cum bene uitaris, tamen auferet; inuenit artem
   femina, qua cupidi carpat amantis opes.                   420
institor ad dominam ueniet discinctus emacem,

---

   395–6 tum (*ita A*ς: tunc *R*³ς) neque te prodet communi noxia (conscia *a*)
culpa / factaque erunt dominae dictaque nota tibi *R*³ (*marg.*) *A*ω: *om. RO,
secl. Merkel*    403 teneras (it̄a *O*) semper tutum *RO*ω: semper tene-
ras tutum *A*ς: teneras tutum semper ς: semper tutum teneras *T*    tutum
*ROA*ω: tutum est ς    413 tum *r*ς: tu *RO, edd.*: tunc *A*ω    414 uul-
neribus latiis *R*ω: u. nostris *AHO*ₐ²: nostris u. *OP*ₐ    416 festa *RA*ς:
sacra *O*ς    syro *R, exc. Put. et Scal.*: uiro *r an R incert., A*ω: deo *O.*
*cf.* 76

    expediet merces teque sedente suas;
quas illa inspicias, sapere ut uideare, rogabit;
    oscula deinde dabit, deinde rogabit emas.
hoc fore contentam multos iurabit in annos;                    425
    nunc opus esse sibi, nunc bene dicet emi.
si non esse domi, quos des, causabere nummos,
    littera poscetur, ne didicisse iuuet.
quid, quasi natali cum poscit munera libo
    et, quotiens opus est, nascitur illa sibi?                 430
quid, cum mendaci damno maestissima plorat
    elapsusque caua fingitur aure lapis?
multa rogant utenda dari, data reddere nolunt;
    perdis, et in damno gratia nulla tuo.
non mihi, sacrilegas meretricum ut persequar artes,           435
    cum totidem linguis sint satis ora decem.
cera uadum temptet rasis infusa tabellis,
    cera tuae primum conscia mentis eat;
blanditias ferat illa tuas imitataque amantum
    uerba, nec exiguas, quisquis es, adde preces.              440
Hectora donauit Priamo prece motus Achilles;
    flectitur iratus uoce rogante deus.
promittas facito, quid enim promittere laedit?
    pollicitis diues quilibet esse potest.
Spes tenet in tempus, semel est si credita, longum;          445
    illa quidem fallax, sed tamen apta, dea est.
si dederis aliquid, poteris ratione relinqui:
    praeteritum tulerit perdideritque nihil.
at quod non dederis, semper uideare daturus:

428 ne ... iuuet *RO* (-bet) *AU* (-uat) $O_gP_c$: nec ... iuuet *aς*: nec ...
iuuat *ω*          433 utenda *ROAbς*: reddenda *aω*          434 tuo *ROς*: tuo
est *Aω*          436 sint *ROς*: sunt *rAω*          438 conscia *RAω*: nuntia
$OP_aW$ (*u.l.*)          439 amantum *RAω*: amoitum *O*: mentem *N*: aman-
tem *Heinsius, Bentleius*          445 tempus ... longum *ROAω*: longum ...
tempus *ςφ*

sic dominum sterilis saepe fefellit ager.                           450
sic, ne perdiderit, non cessat perdere lusor,
   et reuocat cupidas alea saepe manus.
hoc opus, hic labor est, primo sine munere iungi:
   ne dederit gratis quae dedit, usque dabit.
ergo eat et blandis peraretur littera uerbis                         455
   exploretque animos primaque temptet iter:
littera Cydippen pomo perlata fefellit,
   insciaque est uerbis capta puella suis.
disce bonas artes, moneo, Romana iuuentus,
   non tantum trepidos ut tueare reos:                        460
quam populus iudexque grauis lectusque senatus,
   tam dabit eloquio uicta puella manus.
sed lateant uires, nec sis in fronte disertus;
   effugiant uoces uerba molesta tuae.
quis, nisi mentis inops, tenerae declamat amicae?                    465
   saepe ualens odii littera causa fuit.
sit tibi credibilis sermo consuetaque uerba,
   blanda tamen, praesens ut uideare loqui.
si non accipiet scriptum inlectumque remittet,
   lecturam spera propositumque tene.                         470
tempore difficiles ueniunt ad aratra iuuenci,
   tempore lenta pati frena docentur equi.
ferreus adsiduo consumitur anulus usu,
   interit adsidua uomer aduncus humo.
quid magis est saxo durum, quid mollius unda?                        475
   dura tamen molli saxa cauantur aqua.
Penelopen ipsam, persta modo, tempore uinces:
   capta uides sero Pergama, capta tamen.

452 *saepe* $ROA\omega$: blanda $\varsigma\phi$    454 ne $RO$: si $A\omega$    461 lectusque
$Ra\omega$: letusque $OA\varsigma$    463 nec $RA\varsigma$: ne $O\varsigma$    466–71 *om. RO*,
*add. in marg.* r    467 consuetaque $r\varsigma$: consultaque $A\omega$    475–6 *in
pariete Pompeiano scripti* (*C.L.E.* 936. 1–2): 475 quid pote tan durum
saxso aut *eqs.*

legerit et nolit rescribere, cogere noli;

    tu modo blanditias fac legat usque tuas.         480

quae uoluit legisse, uolet rescribere lectis:

    per numeros ueniunt ista gradusque suos.

forsitan et primo uèniet tibi littera tristis

    quaeque roget ne se sollicitare uelis;

quod rogat illa, timet; quod non rogat, optat, ut instes:  485

    insequere, et uoti postmodo compos eris.

interea, siue illa toro resupina feretur,

    lecticam dominae dissimulanter adi;

neue aliquis uerbis odiosas offerat auris,

    qua potes, ambiguis callidus abde notis.        490

seu pedibus uacuis illi spatiosa teretur

    porticus, hic socias tu quoque iunge moras,

et modo praecedas facito, modo terga sequaris,

    et modo festines et modo lentus eas.

nec tibi de mediis aliquot transire columnas       495

    sit pudor aut lateri continuasse latus,

nec sine te curuo sedeat speciosa theatro:

    quod spectes, umeris adferet illa suis.

illam respicias, illam mirere licebit,

    multa supercilio, multa loquare notis;        500

et plaudas aliquam mimo saltante puellam,

    et faueas illi, quisquis agatur amans.

cum surgit, surges; donec sedet illa, sedebis:

---

479 nolit *rAω*: noli *RO*: nolet ς     482 ueniunt *RAωφ*: uenient *O, edd. plerique*     489 offerat *RO*: auferat *W*[1]: efferat *O₉U*: afferat *rAω*: conferat *L*     490 qua *Kenney, F (ut uid.)*: quam *ROAω, edd.* abde *ROAω*: adde ς     495 aliquot *OAω*: aliquod *BU*: aliquid *R*: aliquas ς: aliquam *LP_a*     columnas *ROAς*: columnis ς     497 speciosa *R* (spet-) *OLO₉*: spatiosa *Aω*     499 mirere *Rς*: mirare *OAς* 501 aliquam *Heinsius ex exc. Scal.*: aliqua (mittē *pro* mimo) *O*: aliquo *rAω*: de *R incert.*     puellam *OO₉*: puella *RA (ut uid.)* ς: puelle *raω*     502 et *aω*: ut *ROAς*     503 surgit *ROAς*: surget *bω*     sedebis *ROAς*: sedeto *rbς*

arbitrio dominae tempora perde tuae.
sed tibi nec ferro placeat torquere capillos,            505
    nec tua mordaci pumice crura teras;
ista iube faciant, quorum Cybeleia mater
    concinitur Phrygiis exululata modis.
forma uiros neglecta decet; Minoida Theseus
    abstulit, a nulla tempora comptus acu;           510
Hippolytum Phaedra, nec erat bene cultus, amauit;
    cura deae siluis aptus Adonis erat.
munditie placeant, fuscentur corpora Campo;
    sit bene conueniens et sine labe toga.
†lingua ne rigeat†; careant rubigine dentes;         515
    nec uagus in laxa pes tibi pelle natet;
nec male deformet rigidos tonsura capillos:
    sit coma, sit trita barba resecta manu.
et nihil emineant et sint sine sordibus ungues,
    inque caua nullus stet tibi nare pilus.           520
nec male odorati sit tristis anhelitus oris,
    nec laedat naris uirque paterque gregis.
cetera lasciuae faciant concede puellae
    et si quis male uir quaerit habere uirum.
ecce, suum uatem Liber uocat: hic quoque amantis     525
    adiuuat et flammae, qua calet ipse, fauet.
Cnosis in ignotis amens errabat harenis,
    qua breuis aequoreis Dia feritur aquis;
utque erat e somno, tunica uelata recincta,

---

511 cultus *ROAω*: comptus ς     513 munditie *ROAω, primus edidit*
*Merkel*: munditiae *aP_c, uett. edd.*     515 lingua $RO_a{}^1O_b$ (nec rigeat
lingua): linguam *O*: linguaque *Aω*     ne *ROω*: non *Aς*: nec ς. *varie*
*temptauerunt edd.*; lingula ne rigeat *Goold* (*iam* lingula ne ruget *Palmer*):
gingiuae *latitare credunt A. G. Lee et W. M. Edwards*     518 trita
*Housman*: tuta *RO*: docta *Aω*: scita *Heinsius*     519 et nihil *Itali, $P_b$*:
ut nihil *ROAω*     522 laedat *A* (*ut uid.*) ς: laedant *ROaω*     527 cf.
293     528 dia feritur *Itali, $P_c{}^2$* (*in ras.*): india (insula *N*) fertur *ROAω*

nuda pedem, croceas inreligata comas,                                  530
Thesea crudelem surdas clamabat ad undas,
  indigno teneras imbre rigante genas.
clamabat flebatque simul, sed utrumque decebat;
  non facta est lacrimis turpior illa suis.
iamque iterum tundens mollissima pectora palmis           535
  'perfidus ille abiit: quid mihi fiet?' ait;
'quid mihi fiet?' ait; sonuerunt cymbala toto
  litore et adtonita tympana pulsa manu.
excidit illa metu rupitque nouissima uerba;
  nullus in exanimi corpore sanguis erat.                        540
ecce, Mimallonides sparsis in terga capillis,
  ecce, leues Satyri, praeuia turba dei.
ebrius, ecce, senex pando Silenus asello
  uix sedet et pressas continet arte iubas.
dum sequitur Bacchas, Bacchae fugiuntque petuntque,   545
  quadrupedem ferula dum malus urget eques,
in caput aurito cecidit delapsus asello;
  clamarunt Satyri 'surge age, surge, pater.'
iam deus in curru, quem summum texerat uuis,
  tigribus adiunctis aurea lora dabat;                            550
et color et Theseus et uox abiere puellae,
  terque fugam petiit terque retenta metu est.
horruit, ut steriles agitat quas uentus aristas,
  ut leuis in madida canna palude tremit.
cui deus 'en, adsum tibi cura fidelior' inquit;               555
  'pone metum, Bacchi Cnosias uxor eris.
munus habe caelum: caelo spectabere sidus;
  saepe reget dubiam Cressa Corona ratem.'

---

544 arte *ironice dictum, ne cui adrideat* ante *illud Merkelianum*
553 steriles *uix satis explicatum*     aristas *RO* (-us) *Aς*: aristae ω
556 *cf.* 293     557 caelo *Raω*: caeli *OAς*     558 reget *Y, Merkel ex*
*coni.*: rege *RO*: reges *Aω*

dixit et e curru, ne tigres illa timeret,
    desilit (inposito cessit harena pede)               560
implicitamque sinu, neque enim pugnare ualebat,
    abstulit: in facili est omnia posse deo.
pars 'Hymenaee' canunt, pars clamant 'Euhion, euhoe';
    sic coeunt sacro nupta deusque toro.
ergo, ubi contigerint positi tibi munera Bacchi          565
    atque erit in socii femina parte tori,
Nycteliumque patrem nocturnaque sacra precare
    ne iubeant capiti uina nocere tuo.
hic tibi multa licet sermone latentia tecto
    dicere, quae dici sentiat illa sibi,               570
blanditiasque leues tenui perscribere uino,
    ut dominam in mensa se legat illa tuam,
atque oculos oculis spectare fatentibus ignem:
    saepe tacens uocem uerbaque uultus habet.
fac primus rapias illius tacta labellis            575
    pocula, quaque bibet parte puella, bibas;
et quemcumque cibum digitis libauerit illa,
    tu pete, dumque petes, sit tibi tacta manus.
sint etiam tua uota uiro placuisse puellae:
    utilior uobis factus amicus erit.             580
huic, si sorte bibes, sortem concede priorem,

---

560 pede *ROAω*: pedi ς      562 in facili *R*: ut facili *O$_g$*: en facile
*OP$_a$*[1]: ut facile *Aω*: nam facile *B*: facile (ut *om.*) *φ*    563 hymenaee
*R* (-mine/e) ς: hymenaea *OAω*      canunt *ROω*: uocant *Aς*: uocat ς
pars clamant euchion (*corr. Merkel*) euhoe (*uel sim.*) *R* (e. eluhoe) *O* (euhio
e.) ς: pars clamant eoe (*uel sim.*) bache ς: pars altera clamat ehoe (*uel sim.*)
*A* (*sed* euchion heychoe *sscr. a*) *ω*    571 perscribere *OAω*: p̄scribere
(*i.e.* prae-) *R*: proscribere *B$_b$*    573 oculos oculis *RO* (-us o.) *ω*:
oculis oculos *Aς*    576 bibet *ROAς*: bibit ς: bibat ς    bibas *OAω*:
bibes *Rς*: bibe *B$_b$P$_c$*    577 libauerit *rAς*: librauerit *RO* (-berit) ς
578 petes *Oω*: petis *Abς*: petas *RO$_b$*    580 uobis *Rbω*: uotis *OAς*
581 sorte *Heinsius ex exc. Put. et Scal.*: forte *codd.*    bibes *Aω*: bibas ς:
bibis *O$_g$W*: uides *B$_b$*: tibi *RO*

   huic detur capiti missa corona tuo.
siue erit inferior seu par, prior omnia sumat,
   nec dubites illi uerba secunda loqui.
[tuta frequensque uia est, per amici fallere nomen;     585
   tuta frequensque licet sit uia, crimen habet.
inde procurator nimium quoque multa procurat
   et sibi mandatis plura uidenda putat.]
certa tibi a nobis dabitur mensura bibendi:
   officium praestent mensque pedesque suum.     590
iurgia praecipue uino stimulata caueto
   et nimium faciles ad fera bella manus.
occidit Eurytion stulte data uina bibendo:
   aptior est dulci mensa merumque ioco.
si uox est, canta; si mollia bracchia, salta;     595
   et, quacumque potes dote placere, place.
ebrietas ut uera nocet, sic ficta iuuabit:
   fac titubet blaeso subdola lingua sono,
ut, quicquid facias dicasue proteruius aequo,
   credatur nimium causa fuisse merum.     600
et bene dic dominae, bene, cum quo dormiat illa;
   sed male sit tacita mente precare uiro.
at cum discedet mensa conuiua remota,
   ipsa tibi accessus turba locumque dabit.
insere te turbae leuiterque admotus eunti     605
   uelle latus digitis et pede tange pedem.
conloquii iam tempus adest; fuge rustice longe
   hinc Pudor: audentem Forsque Venusque iuuat.

   583 siue erit ω: siuelit R: si uellit O: siue sit Aς     584 nec ROAω:
ne Aς: neu D     585–8 secl. Weise (587–8 iam Bentleius), hic uix
ferendi sunt. an post 742 ponendi?     585–6 tuta . . . tuta codd.: trita . . .
trita Heinsius     587 procurator ROAω: propinator ς     procurat
ROAω: propinat ς: propinet ς     592 bella Oaωφ: uerba RAς: tela H
608 forsque RO (-ue) AL: sorsque ω: de ς incert.     iuuat ROς: iuuant Aω,
fortasse recte

non tua sub nostras ueniat facundia leges;
   fac tantum cupias, spònte disertus eris.          610
est tibi agendus amans imitandaque uulnera uerbis;
   haec tibi quaeratur qualibet arte fides.
nec credi labor est: sibi quaeque uidetur amanda;
   pessima sit, nulli non sua forma placet.
saepe tamen uere coepit simulator amare;         615
   saepe, quod incipiens finxerat esse, fuit.
(quo magis, o, faciles imitantibus este, puellae:
   fiet amor uerus, qui modo falsus erat.)
blanditiis animum furtim deprendere nunc sit,
   ut pendens liquida ripa subestur aqua.         620
nec faciem nec te pigeat laudare capillos
   et teretes digitos exiguumque pedem:
delectant etiam castas praeconia formae;
   uirginibus curae grataque forma sua est.
nam cur in Phrygiis Iunonem et Pallada siluis     625
   nunc quoque iudicium non tenuisse pudet?
laudatas ostendit auis Iunonia pinnas;
   si tacitus spectes, illa recondit opes.
quadrupedes inter rapidi certamina cursus
   depexaeque iubae plausaque colla iuuant.     630
nec timide promitte: trahunt promissa puellas;
   pollicito testes quoslibet adde deos.
Iuppiter ex alto periuria ridet amantum
   et iubet Aeolios inrita ferre Notos.
per Styga Iunoni falsum iurare solebat        635
   Iuppiter: exemplo nunc fauet ipse suo.

---

  609 ueniat *ROϚ*: ueniet *AϚ*       610 cupias *ROAω*: incipias Ϛ
612 haec *ROAϚ*: hic *ω*: nec *H¹O_g*     619 nunc sit *AϚ*: non sit *ROL²*
(*u.l.*): fas sit Ϛ: fas est *ω*: possit *r*     620 subestur *Axelson*: subetur
*RO*: sudetur *r*: subitur *Aω*: cauatur Ϛ: salitur *L*    627 ostendit
*ROωφ*: ostentat *AϚ*    628 recondit *ROAωφ*: recondet Ϛ    636 ipse
*ROAω*: ille Ϛ

expedit esse deos et, ut expedit, esse putemus;
   dentur in antiquos tura merumque focos.
nec secura quies illos similisque sopori
   detinet: innocue uiuite, numen adest.                              640
reddite depositum; pietas sua foedera seruet;
   fraus absit; uacuas caedis habete manus.
ludite, si sapitis, solas impune puellas:
   †hac magis est una fraude pudenda fides†.
fallite fallentes; ex magna parte profanum                           645
   sunt genus: in laqueos, quos posuere, cadant.
dicitur Aegyptos caruisse iuuantibus arua
   imbribus atque annos sicca fuisse nouem,
cum Thrasius Busirin adit monstratque piari
   hospitis adfuso sanguine posse Iouem.                             650
illi Busiris 'fies Iouis hostia primus'
   inquit 'et Aegypto tu dabis hospes aquam.'
et Phalaris tauro uiolenti membra Perilli
   torruit; infelix inbuit auctor opus.
iustus uterque fuit, neque enim lex aequior ulla est                 655
   quam necis artifices arte perire sua.
ergo, ut periuras merito periuria fallant,
   exemplo doleat femina laesa suo.
et lacrimae prosunt; lacrimis adamanta mouebis:
   fac madidas uideat, si potes, illa genas.                          660
si lacrimae, neque enim ueniunt in tempore semper,
   deficient, uncta lumina tange manu.
quis sapiens blandis non misceat oscula uerbis?
   illa licet non det, non data sume tamen.
pugnabit primo fortassis et 'improbe' dicet;                          665

   644 hac *rOAω*: haec *R*      magis *ROAω*: minus *aς*      fraude *ROAω*:
parte *ς*      pudenda *codd.*: tuenda *Naugerius ex codd., ut ait*: (minus . . .)
tuenda *Burmannus, nescio an recte*          650 adfuso *R*: affuso *O₉*: effuso
*OAω*          662 deficient *RO* (diff-) *Aς*: deficiunt *ς*: deficiant *ς*      uncta
*rAς*: cunta *R*: cuncta *O*: uda *aω*

pugnando uinci se tamen illa uolet.
tantum, ne noceant teneris male rapta labellis
    neue queri possit dura fuisse, caue.
oscula qui sumpsit, si non et cetera sumit,
    haec quoque, quae data sunt, perdere dignus erit.      670
quantum defuerat pleno post oscula uoto?
    ei mihi, rusticitas, non pudor ille fuit.
uim licet appelles: grata est uis ista puellis;
    quod iuuat, inuitae saepe dedisse uolunt.
quaecumque est Veneris subita uiolata rapina,      675
    gaudet, et inprobitas muneris instar habet.
at quae, cum posset cogi, non tacta recessit,
    ut simulet uultu gaudia, tristis erit.
uim passa est Phoebe, uis est allata sorori;
    et gratus raptae raptor uterque fuit.      680
fabula nota quidem, sed non indigna referri,
    Scyrias Haemonio iuncta puella uiro.
iam dea laudatae dederat mala praemia formae
    colle sub Idaeo uincere digna duas;
iam nurus ad Priamum diuerso uenerat orbe,      685
    Graiaque in Iliacis moenibus uxor erat;
iurabant omnes in laesi uerba mariti,
    nam dolor unius publica causa fuit.
turpe, nisi hoc matris precibus tribuisset, Achilles
    ueste uirum longa dissimulatus erat.      690
quid facis, Aeacide? non sunt tua munera lanae;
    tu titulos alia Palladis arte petes.

666 se *ROAω*: sed *ς*      illa *RAω*: ipsa *Oς*      669 sumit *aς*: sumet *D*:
sumat *BOₐ*: sumpsit *ROAω*      670 erit *ROAω*: erat *ς*      673 ap-
pelles *ROa* (*ut uid.*) *ω*: appellet *Aς*      675 subita *OAω*: subito
*Rς*      677 posset *ROaω*: possit *Aς*      679 allata *ROς*: illata *A*
an a incert., *ω*: oblata *F*      683 mala *ROAς*: sua *ς*      684 duas *O*
(*u.l.*) *Pₓ*: uenus *ROAω*      686 graiaque *A* an a incert., *ς*: grataque
*ROω*      692 petes *ω*: petis *R* (*ut uid.*) *OAς*: petas *r* an *R* incert., *TU*:
pete *ς*: feres *Eₐ*: tene *N*

quid tibi cum calathis? clipeo manus apta ferendo est;
   pensa quid in dextra, qua cadet Hector, habes?
reice succinctos operoso stamine fusos:        695
   quassanda est ista Pelias hasta manu.
forte erat in thalamo uirgo regalis eodem;
   haec illum stupro comperit esse uirum.
uiribus illa quidem uicta est (ita credere oportet),
   sed uoluit uinci uiribus illa tamen.        700
saepe 'mane' dixit, cum iam properaret Achilles:
   fortia nam posito sumpserat arma colo.
uis ubi nunc illa est? quid blanda uoce moraris
   auctorem stupri, Deidamia, tui?
scilicet, ut pudor est quaedam coepisse priorem,    705
   sic alio gratum est incipiente pati.
a, nimia est iuueni propriae fiducia formae,
   expectat si quis, dum prior illa roget.
uir prior accedat, uir uerba precantia dicat;
   excipiat blandas comiter illa preces.       710
ut potiare, roga: tantum cupit illa rogari;
   da causam uoti principiumque tui.
Iuppiter ad ueteres supplex heroidas ibat;
   corrupit magnum nulla puella Iouem.
si tamen a precibus tumidos accedere fastus    715
   senseris, incepto parce referque pedem.
quod refugit, multae cupiunt; odere, quod instat:
   lenius instando taedia tolle tui.

693 ferendo *ra* (*ut uid.*) ω: ferenda *RAB*[1] (*ut uid.*) $O_b$: terenda $OO_gP_c$: terendo, gerendo, tenendo, tenenda Ϛ   est *ROaω*: *om. A*Ϛ   702 posito *RO*Ϛ: posita *A*Ϛ   705 quaedam *R*Ϛ: quandam *Oa*Ϛ: quendam *A*Ϛ: quidam *r* (*ut uid.*) $O_a{}^2$ (*ut uid.*): aliquem $P_f$: aliquam *a*: quamquam Ϛ   708 expectat *RA*Ϛ: expectet *O*Ϛ   710 excipiat *ROA*Ϛ: excipiet Ϛ   comiter *RO*: molliter *rA*ω: dulciter $O_bP_f$   714 corrupit *RO* (-rip-) $P_b$: corripuit *rA*ω   715 accedere ω: abscedere *ROA*Ϛ

nec semper Veneris spes est profitenda roganti;
  intret amicitiae nomine tectus amor. 720
hoc aditu uidi tetricae data uerba puellae;
  qui fuerat cultor, factus amator erat.
candidus in nauta turpis color: aequoris unda
  debet et a radiis sideris esse niger;
turpis et agricolae, qui uomere semper adunco 725
  et grauibus rastris sub Ioue uersat humum;
et tua, Palladiae petitur cui fama coronae,
  candida si fuerint corpora, turpis eris.
palleat omnis amans: hic est color aptus amanti;
  hoc decet, hoc multi †non ualuisse† putant. 730
pallidus in Side siluis errabat Orion;
  pallidus in lenta Naide Daphnis erat.
arguat et macies animum, nec turpe putaris
  palliolum nitidis inposuisse comis.
attenuant iuuenum uigilatae corpora noctes 735
  curaque et in magno qui fit amore dolor.
ut uoto potiare tuo, miserabilis esto,
  ut qui te uideat dicere possit 'amas.'
conquerar an moneam mixtum fas omne nefasque?
  nomen amicitia est, nomen inane fides. 740
ei mihi, non tutum est, quod ames, laudare sodali:
  cum tibi laudanti credidit, ipse subit.

---

721 data *ROaς*: dare ς: da *A*     725 qui *aς*: quia *RAς*: quam *O*
727 tua *ROς*: tu *rAω*     fama *ROAω*: palma *Heinsius ex P* b, *edd. ple-
rique*     730 putant *rOAω*: putent *R*     *uersus saepe temptatus*; stulti
. . . putant *Hertzberg, probat Goold*: nulli . . . puta *Hollis (iam* nulli . . .
putent *Mueller)*: multis . . . putas? *Palmer*: multis mox valuisse putant
*dubitanter Kenney*     731 *om. O*     Side *R. Schultze, coll. Apollod. biblioth.*
I iv 3 2 (*Sides mentionem iam fecerat Heinsius*): linces *R*: linchas *O*g: linca
*rAω*: lincem, licea, licien, licita, lotica ς     orion *aω*: arion *RA* (*ut uid.*),
*Schol. Haun.*     734 palliolum *ROAς*: pilliolum ς     739 omne
*ROAςφ*: esse ς     741 ames *ROabς*: amas *Aς*

'at non Actorides lectum temerauit Achillis;
　　quantum ad Pirithoum, Phaedra pudica fuit.
Hermionen Pylades, qua Pallada Phoebus, amabat,               745
　　quodque tibi geminus, Tyndari, Castor, erat.'
si quis idem sperat, iacturas poma myricas
　　speret et e medio flumine mella petat.
nil nisi turpe iuuat; curae sua cuique uoluptas;
　　haec quoque ab alterius grata dolore uenit.               750
heu facinus, non est hostis metuendus amanti;
　　quos credis fidos, effuge: tutus eris.
cognatum fratremque caue carumque sodalem;
　　praebebit ueros haec tibi turba metus.
finiturus eram, sed sunt diuersa puellis                      755
　　pectora; mille animos excipe mille modis.
nec tellus eadem parit omnia: uitibus illa
　　conuenit, haec oleis; hic bene farra uirent.
pectoribus mores tot sunt, quot in ore figurae:
　　qui sapit, innumeris moribus aptus erit,                  760
utque leues Proteus modo se tenuabit in undas,
　　nunc leo, nunc arbor, nunc erit hirtus aper.
hi iaculo pisces, illi capiuntur ab hamis,
　　hos caua contento retia fune trahunt:
nec tibi conueniet cunctos modus unus ad annos;              765
　　longius insidias cerua uidebit anus.
si doctus uideare rudi petulansue pudenti,
　　diffidet miserae protinus illa sibi.

745 hermionen *OAꝗ*: hermionem *R* (*ut uid.*) *ω*: hermionam *r*, *edd.*
qua *Madvig* (*coll.* i 285), *U*: quo *aω*: quod *ROA*　　amabat *RO* (-uat)
*Aꝗ*: amauit *ꝗ*　　746 quodque *ROA* (*ut uid.*) *ω*: quoque *aꝗ*: quaque *U*
747 iacturas *ROAꝗ, nescio an recte*: laturas *raω*　　748 e *ROAꝗ*: in *ꝗ*
759 ore *Bentleius*: orbe *ROAωφ, edd.*　　761 leues *ROAꝗ*: leuis *ω*
modo se *ROaω*: sese *Aꝗ*: corpus *D*　　tenuabit *Itali*: tenuauit *Rꝗ*: tenua-
bat *OAω*　　762 erit *RO*: erat *Aω*　　763 hi *rAꝗ*: hic *ROωφ*
illi *Aꝗ*: illic *Oωφ*: illa *R*　　764 hos *Aω*: hic *rꝗφ*: hoc *R*: haec *O*
766 cerua *RO* (*u.l.*): curua *rOAω*

inde fit ut, quae se timuit committere honesto,
uilis ad amplexus inferioris eat.

770

Pars superat coepti, pars est exhausta, laboris;
hic teneat nostras ancora iacta rates.

---

770 ad *RAω*: in *O*ϛ          771 superat *ROA* (*ut uid.*) ϛ: superest *aω*
P. OVIDII NASONIS ARTIS AMATORIAE LIBER PRIMVS EXPR;IMτ (RIM *in ras.*,
*nota* ';' *a r addita; de* 'τ' *incert.*) *R*

# COMMENTARY

**1–34.** *Prologue*

Ovid starts with a paradox—there is a skill of love which can be communicated by teaching. No one would deny that steering a ship or driving a chariot requires skill, and the same is true of love (3–4). Furthermore there must be one man in charge of each operation; for this part Ovid has unique qualifications, having been entrusted by Venus with the education of her son, Cupid (5–8). The boy proves a difficult pupil, but Chiron succeeded in taming the equally troublesome Achilles (9–24). This work springs from the author's personal experience; he makes no claim to be supernaturally inspired (25–30). The poem is not directed at respectable Roman matrons, and thus will be found to contain nothing objectionable or illegal (31–4).

This prologue is chiefly distinguished by elegant and unexpected variation of stock themes (17, 21) and some ingenious literary polemic (25–30).

**1–2.** A confident assertion of the poem's value and the benefits which it will confer, addressed not, as in many didactic works, to a named individual (e.g. Perses, Memmius) but to every Roman who is ignorant of the art of love. At once Ovid makes plain that he will write for the context of the capital city, not in the half-Greek, half-Roman world traditional to Latin elegy. Such Roman colouring is particularly noticeable in book i, and in my opinion provides one of the greatest charms of the *Ars*.

**1. in hoc . . . populo :** cf. Cicero, *de Or.* ii. 153 'probabiliorem huic populo oratorem'. A commoner phrase for the Roman people would be 'in tanto populo' (Nisbet on Cic., *in Pisonem* 95. 13).

**Si quis . . . artem . . . non nouit amandi** : A didactic poet is likely to emphasize the pitiable state of those ignorant of his art. Conceivably Ovid echoes Virgil's statement that he undertook the *Georgics* through pity for the 'ignaros . . . uiae . . . agrestis' (i. 41); cf. also Grattius, *Cynegetica* i. 98, the inventor of hunting equipment 'ignarum perfudit lumine uolgus' and for the wording Moschus, fr. 2. 7 Gow ταῦτα λέγω πᾶσιν τὰ διδάγματα τοῖς ἀνεράστοις ('I give this advice to all those who have not experienced love'). The notorious treatise περὶ ἀφροδισίων (fragments preserved in *P. Oxy.* vol. 39 (1972), no. 2891) started something like 'Philaenis compiled this work for those desiring . . . (? to lead a life of pleasure)'.

**artem . . . amandi** : the nearest approach to the poem's title that dactylic verse will allow. In fact some early editors entitled

the work *de Arte Amandi*, but *Ars Amatoria* is supported
by ancient evidence, e.g. Seneca, *Contr.* iii. 7 'hoc saeculum
*amatoriis* non *artibus* tantum sed sententiis impleuit.'

'Ars' is the key-word, appearing early and often repeated.
Similarly Grattius begins his work on hunting 'Dona cano
diuom, laetas uenantibus *artis*' and constantly returns to the
noun 'ars', making a contrast with the primitive age when man
hunted 'nuda . . . uirtute' (3) and even notable figures like
Adonis who tangled with the beasts 'meo sine munere' (65)
came to grief. The Greek counterpart is of course τέχνη, e.g.
Oppian, *Halieutica* iii. 1–2 νῦν δ᾽ ἄγε μοι, σκηπτοῦχε, παναίολα δήνεα
τέχνης / ἰχθυβόλου φράζοιο.

**2. hoc legat :** H. Tränkle (*Hermes* 100 (1972), 388–90) would
revive the variant 'me legat' (read also by Y). But the switch
'*me* legat . . . lecto *carmine*', though accepted by some good
scholars in the past, seems hardly tolerable. The variant might
be ancient; in an imitation at *Anth. Lat.* 674a. 1–2 Riese
'Maeonium quisquis Romanus nescit Homerum / me legat et
lectum credat utrumque sibi' the same awkwardness does not,
however, occur.

**3–4.** The threefold 'arte' binds together the argument; we cannot
question Ovid's first two propositions, and so accept the third.
The epithets applied to ships and chariots, 'citae' and 'leues',
gain in point because mobility and fickleness are notorious
qualities of that Love whom Ovid must control.

**5. Automedon :** the charioteer of Achilles. He became semi-
proverbial (cf. 8), like Jehu—Cicero, *pro Sex. Roscio* 98 'Auto-
medontem illum', Juvenal 1. 61.

**6. Tiphys :** helmsman of the Argo in the best-known versions.

**7 ff.** The author has been appointed by Venus herself as tutor to
Cupid. This is an unexpected idea, reaching its climax at 17 'ego
sum praeceptor Amoris', but it does not prove very fruitful and is
soon abandoned thereafter. Ovid may be influenced by a piece
of the bucolic poet Bion (*c.* 100 B.C.), fr. 10 Gow (quoted with
Cowper's translation in my Appendix II): Aphrodite in a dream
asks the poet to teach Eros music, but the boy pays no attention
and instead teaches Bion about love (cf. Ovid lines 21–4).

**10. aetas :** in apposition to *puer* ('an age tender and open to
guidance'), cf. *Met.* iii. 540–1 'uosne, acrior aetas, / o iuuenes'.

**11 ff.** The centaur Chiron (Phillyrides), who was particularly
skilled in music and medicine, educated several young men of
noble or semi-divine birth, among them Achilles. A poem current
in antiquity and ascribed to Hesiod (Χείρωνος ὑποθῆκαι, frs.
283–5 Merkelbach–West) purported to contain the lessons given
to Achilles by Chiron. Also a nice Pompeian wall-painting
(illustrated in Roscher s.v. Cheiron) shows Chiron, Achilles, and

the lyre. Can one detect a meek and apprehensive look on Achilles' face (cf. 14, 16 n.)?

**11. cithara perfecit**: 'made him accomplished in lyre-playing'.

**12. placida contudit arte**: an effective word-order, since by itself the verb would imply a violent subjection.

**13. socios**: because the wrath of Achilles caused innumerable sufferings to his fellow Greeks (*Iliad* i. 1–2).

**15–16. quas Hector sensurus erat . . . / . . . manus**: Homer more than once mentions the 'man-slaying hands' of Achilles—Ovid may have in mind chiefly *Iliad* xxiv. 478–9 where Priam, hoping to ransom the body of Hector, kisses Achilles' hands δεινὰς ἀνδροφόνους, αἵ οἱ πολέας κτάνον υἷας.

**15. sensurus**: The menacing understatement is also Homeric, *Iliad* xviii. 269–70 (Hector on Achilles) εὖ νύ τις αὐτὸν / γνώσεται (cf. Horace, *Odes* i. 15. 26–7 'Merionen quoque / nosces').

**16.** Juvenal has a similar picture, 'metuens uirgae iam grandis Achilles' (7. 210). Chiron is made into a grim Roman school-master, like Horace's 'plagosus' Orbilius (*Epist.* ii. 1. 70); cf. Juvenal i. 15 'et nos ergo manum ferulae subduximus.'

    **iussas**: in effect 'as ordered', cf. *Met.* i. 399 'iussos lapides sua post uestigia mittunt.'

**17. praeceptor Amoris**: These words represent the whole work at *Tristia* i. 1. 67 '"inspice" dic "titulum. non sum praeceptor amoris."' We expect them to mean 'a teacher of love', as ii. 161 'praeceptor amandi', *Fasti* vi. 13 (of Hesiod) 'praeceptor arandi'. So it is a surprise that Ovid means here 'the tutor of Cupid'. A play on two levels by which 'amoris' = at once love and Cupid (see on 231–6) would be unwelcome, since 'Amoris' must balance 'Aeacidae' and both be picked up by 'uterque puer' (18). But of course nothing prevented Ovid from repeating the phrase in its natural sense (*Tristia* i. 1. 67 above, cf. *A.A.* ii. 497); without these echoes one might be tempted by the old conjecture 'Amori'. For the poet as teacher of Cupid see on 7 ff. and Appendix II. The image is virtually abandoned by line 24, but Ovid returns to it poignantly in exile (*ex Ponto* iii. 3 e.g. line 46 'discipulo perii solus ab ipse meo').

**18. saeuus uterque puer, natus uterque dea**: typical of our poet's rhetorically trained mind, which was quick to spot the similarities in apparently disparate examples. The famous comparison of a lover and a soldier ('militat omnis amans', *Amores* i. 9) shows the same technique on a larger scale.

    Note that the two halves of the pentameter are metrically interchangeable, both ending in a disyllable. This happens seldom (Platnauer, *Latin Elegiac Verse*, pp. 14–15), and usually with some repetition of words, as here; cf. the notorious 'semi-bouemque uirum, semiuirumque bouem' (ii. 24).

**19–20.** The breaking-in of cattle and horses, as with most of Ovid's countryside images, can be found also in Virgil's *Georgics* (iii. 163 ff., 179 ff.). Thus the examples gain a little more life by reminding us that the *Ars* is a didactic poem. A much more striking instance occurs in 93–6; see generally Eleanor Leach, 'Georgic Imagery in the *Ars Amatoria*', *TAPA* 95 (1964), 142–54.

**20. frenaque magnanimi dente teruntur equi :** He presents the hackneyed illustration in an unusual way. Of course the point lies in the taming of a spirited horse, not in the gradual wearing away of metal (a regular example of how persistence can achieve results, e.g. 473–4). Therefore the force of 'teruntur' must be that, once having submitted to the bridle, the horse is never free from it (cf. Horace, *Epist.* i. 10. 38).

  **magnanimi :** an epithet belonging to the high epic style (cf. μεγάθυμος) which may derive from Ennius.

**21. et mihi cedet Amor :** surely an intentional reversal of Virgil's 'omnia uincit Amor, *et nos cedamus Amori*' (*Ecl.* 10. 69).

**22. excutiatque :** 'brandishes' (meaning no more than the simple 'quatio', as at 235). His purpose is to keep the torch burning brightly—thus *Amores* i. 2. 11–12 'uidi ego iactatas mota face crescere flammas / et uidi nullo concutiente mori.' Anyone within range is at risk (cf. 236).

**24. ultor :** by revealing Cupid's secrets and so breaking his power over mankind.

**25–30.** W. Suerbaum (*Hermes* 93 (1965), 491–6) examines these lines in detail, and F. W. Lenz more generally (*Maia* 13 (1961), 131–42 = *Opuscula Selecta* (Amsterdam, 1972), 261–72), but they both leave some tricks to be taken.

  Ovid relies on readers having a considerable knowledge of Greek poetry, both archaic and Alexandrian with its Roman followers (in fact much Alexandrian literary theorizing derived from Hesiod and early lyric). Poets often claimed to have received a supernatural initiation in their art—they met the Muses, were presented with the pipes of Hesiod, conversed with Apollo or the ghost of Homer, or drank from Hippocrene. Their object was to show the high quality of their inspiration, and the absolute veracity of their subject-matter. To aid the latter impression they often presented themselves as passing on information from a superior being (a god or Muse) to their readers, so that the poet became just a passive intermediary. This attitude may be exemplified by Callimachus, *hymn* 3. 186 εἰπέ, θεή, σὺ μὲν ἄμμιν, ἐγὼ δ' ἑτέροισιν ἀείσω ('Goddess, you tell me, and I will sing to the others'—see further on 27–8).

  Also there were notorious cases of Hellenistic poets who had no personal knowledge of their subject, but composed in a bookish way, usually by versifying some prose treatise. Aratus was ignorant of astronomy ('hominem ignarum astrologiae', Cicero, *de Or.* i. 69), but, relying on a treatise by Eudoxus, could write *Phaenomena*, while Nicander of Colophon never poked his nose outside the library (ibid., 'hominem ab agro remotissimum') and yet he composed passable *Georgica*. Ovid's own position is quite different—'usus opus mouet hoc: uati parete perito' (29). There is a certain irony, no doubt intentional, in Ovid rejecting the learned tradition to which he owed so much. But Propertius, whose debt to Alexandria was equally great, and who elsewhere wrote a conventional initiation-poem (iii. 3), could say of his love-poetry addressed to Cynthia (ii. 1. 3–4)

> non haec Calliope, non haec mihi cantat Apollo;
> ingenium nobis ipsa puella facit.

Interesting too is the Prologue (lines 1–6) of the Neronian satirist Persius:

> Nec fonte labra prolui caballino
> nec in bicipiti somniasse Parnaso
> memini, ut repente sic poeta prodirem
> Heliconidasque pallidamque Pirenen
> illis remitto quorum imagines lambunt
> hederae sequaces.

Persius' scholiast tells us that the satirist aims particularly at Ennius; for the vexed problem of the initiation in *Annals* bk. i, see O. Skutsch, *Studia Enniana*, pp. 119–29 (with reference to earlier views). Christian poets later took up this rejection of pagan symbols (see W. Wimmel, *Kallimachos in Rom*, pp. 310–11).

**25. non ego, Phoebe, datas a te mihi mentiar artes :** The main target is Callimachus, who originated this *topos* in the Prologue to his *Aetia*, fr. 1. 22 ff. καὶ γὰρ ὅτε πρώτιστον ἐμοῖς ἐπὶ δέλτον ἔθηκα / γούνασιν, Ἀπόλλων εἶπεν ὅ μοι Λύκιος ('for when first I put the tablet upon my knees, Lycian Apollo said to me . . .'). In the *Aetia* Apollo warned the writer against unsuitable styles and subjects (similarly Virgil, *Ecl.* 6. 3 ff., Propertius iii. 3. 13 ff., Horace, *Odes* iv. 15. 1 ff.); for him actually communicating poetry cf. Propertius ii. 1. 3 (quoted above) and iv. 1. 133 'tum tibi pauca suo de carmine dictat Apollo.'

   **datas a te mihi :** Should we imagine Apollo handing over a complete work, or the poet taking down word for word from the god's dictation as in Prop. iv. 1. 133 (above)?

   **mentiar :** corrected by 'uera canam' (30, see note there).

   **artes :** probably 'my *Ars*'. For the plural cf. *Remedia* 487 'artes tu perlege nostras', *ex Ponto* i. 1. 12.

**26. nec nos aeriae uoce monemur auis :** To balance the allusions in
25 and 27–8 we must look for cases of a poet being inspired by
the birds. This seems to have been a widespread notion (Athe-
naeus ix. 390a quoting Chamaeleon of Pontus), e.g. Aristophanes,
*Birds* 749–50 on Phrynichus, Theophilus of Antioch *ad Auto-
lycum* ii. 30 on Orpheus (see further Bailey on Lucretius v.
1379). If Ovid has a single figure in mind, I suggest that it is
the lyric poet Alcman. Besides being conversant with birds in
general (*Lyrica Graeca Selecta* (Page), 14 ϝοῖδα δ᾽ ὀρνίχων νόμως /
πάντων), Alcman acknowledged a specific debt to the partridges
(ibid. 13 ϝέπη τάδε καὶ μέλος Ἀλκμὰν / εὗρε γεγλωσσαμέναν / κακκαβίδων
ὄπα συνθέμενος); as in Ovid the implication may be that he learned
his subject-matter as well as his art from them.

    In fact D. Korzeniewski (*Hermes* 92 (1964), 200 n. 2) mentions
Alcman, together with two interesting passages on Stesichorus
(*Anth. Pal.* ii. 128–30, Pliny *N.H.* x. 82), but then alights less
happily on Ennius' peacock. For other attempts to explain the
line (none of them really providing the essential point) see
H. Tränkle, *Hermes* 1972, 390–1.

    **monemur :** 'am I prompted', cf. *Aeneid* vii. 41 'tu uatem, tu,
diua, mone' (similarly of giving factual information).

**27–8. nec mihi sunt uisae Clio Cliusque sorores / seruanti pecudes
uallibus, Ascra, tuis :** Ascra, the Boeotian village where Hesiod
lived (*Works and Days* 639–40), points us to *Theogony* 22–34
and the encounter wherein the Muses granted Hesiod the gift of
song (22) together with a staff and knowledge of the past and
future (30–2). M. L. West (ad loc.) has an interesting note on
such visitations.

    No less celebrated (and also no doubt in our poet's mind) was
the original prologue to Callimachus' *Aetia* (fr. 2) which looked
back to Hesiod (lines 1–2 ποιμένι μῆλα νέμοντι παρ᾽ ἴχνιον ὀξέος
ἵππου / ʽΗσιόδῳ Μουσέων ἑσμὸς ὅτ᾽ ἠντίασεν) and related how Calli-
machus too met the Muses—though in a dream, not while
tending sheep. In the earlier parts of the *Aetia* Callimachus
asked the Muses factual questions (e.g. 'Who was the mother of
the Graces?') and was given the answer by individual Muses
speaking in turn, so that the poet became merely an intermedi-
ary between the Muses and his readers. Such a bald summary
may make the *Aetia* sound dull, but it was full of life and had an
attractive dry humour.

**27. Clio Cliusque sorores :** Hesiod does not single out any individual
Muse, but in Callimachus Clio first spoke to the poet followed by
several of her sisters (see *Schol. Flor.*, Pfeiffer vol. I, p. 13 line 30
and on fr. 43. 56, with *P. Ant.* 113 fr. 1ᵃ. 8 adding Erato).

**28. seruanti pecudes :** cf. Hesiod, *Theogony* 23 ἄρνας ποιμαίνονθ᾽
ʽΕλικῶνος ὑπὸ ζαθέοιο ('as he was shepherding his lambs under

holy Helicon'), and Callimachus on Hesiod (fr. 2. 1 quoted
above).

**29. usus opus mouet hoc :** unlike Aratus and Nicander (see on 25–
30). As a factual statement of how Ovid conducted his life, this
must of course be taken with a pinch of salt. Contrast *Tristia* ii.
349 ff., particularly 355–6 'magnaque pars mendax operum est
et ficta meorum : / plus sibi permisit compositore suo.' Personal
immorality did not form part of the indictment against Ovid.
'Usus', 'Experience', is almost personified here, and may
stretch beyond the author's experience. Compare Lucretius v.
1452–3 'usus et impigrae simul experientia mentis / paulatim
docuit pedetemptim progredientis', Virgil, *Georgics* i. 133 'ut
uarias usus meditando extunderet artis'.

**mouet :** grandiose (like ἐγείρω in Greek), cf. *Aeneid* vii. 45
'maius opus moueo.'

**parete perito :** cf. Propertius i. 9. 7 'me dolor et lacrimae merito
fecere peritum.' Most Roman poets would have considered the
jingle a positive adornment ; as e.g. Ennius, *Medea* 260 Warming-
ton 'era errans', Virgil, *Aeneid* iii. 540 'armantur . . . armenta
minantur', iv. 238 'parere parabat', vi. 204 'auri . . . aura' (see
further Norden ad loc.).

**30. uera canam :** echoing now Hesiod's Prologue to the *Works
and Days*, 10 ἐγὼ δέ κε, Πέρση, ἐτήτυμα μυθησαίμην ('and I, Perses,
would tell what is true', cf. West on *Theogony* 26–8). Poets
did not have an invariable reputation for truthfulness—πολλὰ
ψεύδονται ἀοιδοί (Solon fr. 29 West).

**coeptis, mater Amoris, ades :** naturally—as Virgil invokes the
country gods (*Georgics* i. 5 ff.), Grattius Diana (*Cynegetica* 2)
and Oppian Neptune (*Halieutica* i. 73–4).

**31–4.** We must remember that in 18 B.C. adultery had become
a criminal offence with severe penalties under the *Lex Iulia de
adulteriis coercendis* (see Owen on *Tristia* ii. 346); thereafter the
love-poet might find himself in an awkward position. Clearly
Ovid laid great stress on these four lines, to avert any charge
that he was encouraging married women to be unfaithful.
When the charge was in fact made (*Tristia* ii. 212, 346) he con-
stantly refers to this passage as proving his innocence; at
*Tristia* ii. 247–50 the lines are quoted with the substitution of
'nil nisi legitimum' for 'nos Venerem tutam', cf. also *Tristia* ii.
303–4 and *ex Ponto* iii. 3. 51–2.

**31–2. este procul, uittae tenues, insigne pudoris, / quaeque tegis
medios instita longa pedes :** The message is that respectable
married women (matronae) should not read the *Ars*; for similar
prohibitions cf. *Amores* ii. 1. 3 ff., Martial iii. 68, *Priapea* 8. 1–2
'matronae procul hinc abite castae : / turpe est uos legere

impudica uerba.' At *Tristia* ii. 303 Ovid points to this passage
as showing that the work was composed 'solis meretricibus'. On
the involved and somewhat unreal question concerning the status
of young women in the *Ars*, see further Introduction pp. xv–xvii.
Both items of dress in this couplet (hair-band and long skirt) are
mentioned by Tibullus, i. 6. 67–8, speaking of Delia:

> sit modo casta, doce, quamuis non uitta ligatos
>     impediat crines nec stola longa pedes.

Scholars regularly conclude that Delia must have been a *mere-
trix*, but for a different view see Gordon Williams, *Tradition and
Originality in Roman Poetry*, pp. 536–7.

**31. este procul :** a ritual cry. The poet has invoked Venus (30), and
now he must order off any unqualified person whose presence
might vitiate the ceremony. Thus Callimachus, *hymn* 2. 2 ἑκὰς
ἑκὰς ὅστις ἀλιτρός and *Aeneid* vi. 258 'procul o, procul este
profani.' Of course Ovids' address to Venus has been perfunc-
tory, and he makes no attempt to build up the excitement of
a divine epiphany like Callimachus or Virgil. Our poet later
argued in similar terms that he was not responsible if anyone
disregarded the prohibition: 'quaecumque erupit qua non sinit
ire sacerdos / protinus huic dempti criminis ipsa rea est' (*Tristia*
ii. 305–6, see Owen ad loc.).

    **uittae tenues :** These were bands, normally of wool, about the
width of an index finger, which were wound round the head and
tied in a knot at the back of the neck (Lillian M. Wilson, *The
Clothing of the Ancient Romans* (Johns Hopkins Press, 1938),
pp. 140–1 on the *uittae* of Vestals, also her figs. 92a and b). Above
all they characterized Roman matrons; indeed Servius on *Aeneid*
vii. 403 says 'solarum matronarum erant, nam meretricibus non
dabantur.' In fact both Vestal Virgins and unmarried free-born
girls (ingenuae) wore *uittae*, perhaps of a slightly different form
(cf. Prop. iv. 11. 34, Cornelia on her marriage, 'uinxit et ac-
ceptas altera uitta comas'). But the important point is that
they were denied to *meretrices*.

**32. instita longa :** The proper dress of a Roman matron was the
*stola*, which reached almost to the ground and covered the feet
(Lillian Wilson, p. 156 with sculptured figures of matrons nos.
85, 96, 97). But writers often single out the *instita* and make it
stand for the whole *stola*, as here (with the epithet *longa*) and at
ii. 600 'in nostris instita nulla iocis'. No clear representation of
the *instita* seems to have survived in Roman art (Wilson, p. 157),
but the literary sources make it plain enough that this was
a band sewed on to the lower edge of a matron's dress. Compare
particularly Horace, *Satires* i. 2. 29 (matrons) 'quarum subsuta
talos tegat instita ueste'.

**medios . . . pedes :** because the long *stola* cut the feet in half, leaving only the front part exposed.

**33. Venerem tutam :** cf. Horace, *Sat.* i. 2. 47–8 'tutior at quanto merx est in classe secunda, / libertinarum dico', and for 'concessa . . . furta', *Sat.* i. 4. 113–14 'ne sequerer moechas, concessa cum Venere uti / possem'.

**35–40.** *Summary of Proposed Contents.* (A) 35–6, *How to find your girl* (covering i. 41–262) (B) 37, *How to win her favours* (covering i. 269–770) (C) 38, *How to keep her love* (covering book ii). Such a summary is quite in the didactic manner. Consider *Georgics* i. 1–5 'Quid faciat laetas segetes, quo sidere terram / uertere, Maecenas (so far book i), ulmisque adiungere uites (bk. ii) / conueniat, quae cura boum, qui cultus habendo / sit pecori (bk. iii), apibus quanta experientia parcis (bk. iv) / hinc canere incipiam.' Also Lucretius i. 54–61 contains a synopsis (though a less full one) of the main themes to follow—see Bailey's notes. From the Greek one can add Nicander, *Theriaca* 1 ff., 493 ff. A related feature is the recapitulation telling us how far we have progressed in the argument (263 ff., cf. *Georgics* ii. 1 ff.).

It will be noticed that Ovid makes no mention of bk. iii, in which he tells young women how to deal with their male admirers (similarly at 771). Originally he planned only two books, and did not trouble to change these passages (see further Introduction pp. xii–xiii).

**35. Principio :** a favourite way to introduce the first stage of an argument in Lucretius and Virgil's *Georgics* (cf. Kenney in *Ovidiana*, p. 202). Traditional didactic language is found most frequently in Ovid's transitions and introductions.

**quod amare uelis :** 'an appropriate object for your love', affecting the dry and unemotional tone of a technical treatise, like 'materiam . . . amori' (49).

**reperire labora :** picked up by 'labor' in 37. One may see here an echo of Virgil's assertion (deriving from Hesiod) that constant hard work is necessary in agriculture, 'labor omnia uincit' (*Georgics* i. 145). See further Eleanor Leach, *TAPA* 1964, 150–1. I wonder whether 'principio . . . labora, proximus . . . labor, tertius . . .' contain a side-reference to the labours of Hercules. Then 'hic modus' (39) would have more edge: you need only perform three labours, not twelve (compare Plautus, *Persa* 1 ff.).

**36. qui noua nunc primum miles in arma uenis :** no previous experience required. Bishop Theodulf of Orleans (Migne, *Patrologia Latina* vol. 105, col. 312) borrowed the line (with *uenit* for *uenis*) and applied it to the monastic life—Ovid would have liked that.

The image of the lover as a soldier finds its most celebrated expression in *Amores* i. 9, but was firmly established before then, e.g. Horace, *Odes* iii. 26. 1–2 'Vixi puellis nuper idoneus / et militaui non sine gloria.' In Greek notable is fr. 234 Edmonds of the Middle Comedy poet Alexis, which also refers to love's labour: τίς οὐχὶ φήσει τοὺς ἐρῶντας ζῆν πόνοις, / εἰ δεῖ γε πρῶτον μὲν στρατευτικωτάτους / εἶναι, πονεῖν τε δυναμένους τοῖς σώμασι | μάλιστα κτλ. ('Who will deny that a lover's life involves hard work? First of all he must be very much like a soldier, and capable of the utmost physical labour . . .').

**39–40.** Compare Propertius iv. 1. 69–70 'sacra diesque canam et cognomina prisca locorum: / has meus ad metas sudet oportet equus.' The two standard figures in the *Ars* for the poet's progress in his task are a chariot and a ship (e.g. 772); see Kenney in *Ovidiana*, pp. 205–6. Both occur in Pindar and other early lyricists (see Bowra, *Pindar*, p. 230). From there the chariot image passed to Choerilus of Samos (*c*. 450 B.C.). Bewailing his position as an epic poet born too late, Choerilus likened himself to the back-marker in a chariot-race: ὕστατοι ὥστε δρόμου καταλείπομεθ', οὐδέ πῃ ἔστι / πάντῃ παπταίνοντα νεοζυγὲς ἅρμα πελάσσαι (fr. 1. 4–5 Kinkel). But it was Callimachus (fr. 1. 25–8) who bequeathed the figure to his Roman followers.

**39. haec nostro signabitur area curru** : adapted from the Roman custom of driving a plough round the site of a future city, cf. *Fasti* iv. 819 'apta dies legitur qua moenia signet aratro' and Frazer ad loc. So the poet is marking out the bounds of his subject-matter.

**area** : properly a space unoccupied by buildings (helping the metaphor described above). For its use of a poetic field cf. *Amores* iii. 1. 26 and iii. 15. 18.

**40. haec erit admissa meta premenda rota** : According to Kenney (in *Ovidiana*, p. 206 n. 8) 'The couplet ought to mean, simply, "this is as far as I shall go": the addition of the pentameter, which implies that the *speed* of rounding the *meta* is important, spoils it.' The explanation may be that the chariot-motif sometimes appears as a race between the poet and his rivals—cf. Choerilus quoted above and Propertius iii. 1. 13 'quid frustra missis in me certatis habenis?'

**admissa . . . rota** : 'with speeding wheels', cf. *Met.* i. 532 'admisso . . . passu'. The expression seems to derive from 'admittere (or immittere) equum', to give free rein to a horse.

**premenda** : There is little to choose between this and the variant 'terenda' (as e.g. Prop. ii. 25. 26 'septima quam metam triuerit ante rota'). G. P. Goold, *Harvard Studies in Classical Philology* 69 (1965), 60 appears to argue that 'terenda' must be right because 'premere' can only mean 'to press from above', but cf. Horace, *Odes* ii. 10. 3–4 'nimium premendo / litus iniquum' (Licinius hardly contemplated travelling by aeroplane). Of course the charioteer had almost to graze the *meta* as he passed; to round it in a wide arc showed gross incompetence, and one ran the risk of being overtaken on the inside (*Amores* iii. 2. 69–70).

**41–66.** *First you must find a girl. She will not fall into your lap as a gift from the gods ; you must go out and look for her. That involves getting to know the places where females congregate. No need to go abroad—your native Rome will provide all that you can desire in quality, number, and variety.*

**42. elige cui dicas 'tu mihi sola places' :** a delightful combination of the two concepts of love (see further Introduction p. xviii). On the one hand 'elige' suggests cool, rational choice after surveying the whole field, while 'sola' implies that you have no say in the matter. But notice 'dum licet' (41); there may come a time when you are really in love and no longer a free agent.

**'tu mihi sola places' :** the typical declaration of an elegiac lover. These same words are found also at Propertius ii. 7. 19 and [Tibullus] iii. 19 (= iv. 13). 3.

**43. delapsa per auras :** a proverbial expression (Otto, *Die Sprichwörter der Römer* s.v. *Caelum* 8; cf. Headlam on Herodas 1. 9) which betokens not only the miraculous and unexpected arrival of the wonderful gift from heaven (Cicero, *de Imp. Cn. Pomp.* 41 'Cn. Pompeium sicut aliquem . . . de caelo delapsum intuentur', Tibullus i. 3. 90 'sed uidear caelo missus adesse tibi') but also that the recipient has done nothing to earn it (Livy vii. 12. 13 'qui nihil agenti sibi de caelo deuolaturam in sinum uictoriam censeat'). Compare [Tibullus] iii. 19 (= iv. 13). 13 'nunc licet e caelo mittatur amica Tibullo'.

**45–8.** Stereotyped illustrations, which may seem dull but contain more than meets the eye. Hunting, fowling, and fishing were established images in erotic poetry for love's pursuit and capture (Kenney, *Mnemosyne* 23 (1970), 386–8 gives examples). At the same time Ovid likes to draw his analogies from regular subjects of didactic literature (see on 19–20)—these would be *Cynegetica, Ixeutica,* and *Halieutica* respectively (see A. W. Mair's Loeb *Oppian,* pp. xxxii–xlviii)—and to suggest that love is quite as worthy and strenuous an occupation as e.g. hunting.

**49. materiam . . . amori :** The phrase has a somewhat dry and unemotional quality (cf. Horace, *Ars Poetica* 38–9 'sumite materiam uestris, qui scribitis, aequam / uiribus'). Elsewhere the girl may be described as material for love-poetry (*Amores* i. 1. 19, i. 3. 19 'te mihi materiem felicem in carmina praebe').

**50. ante frequens quo sit disce puella loco :** We would expect a work
on hunting to start by talking of the beast's lair, as [Oppian],
*Cyn.* iv. 79 ff. (lion-hunters) χῶρον μὲν πρώτιστον ἐπεφράσσαντο κιόντες.

    **ante . . . disce :** another didactic touch—the manifold pre-
paration necessary before one can undertake the main task.
Thus e.g. *Georgics* i. 50 ff. 'at prius ignotum ferro quam scindi-
mus aequor / uentos et uarium caeli praediscere morem / cura
sit', Lucretius v. 110, Manilius i. 809.

    **puella :** The collective, like 'multo pisce' (48), is hunting lan-
guage. Nisbet and Hubbard on Horace, *Odes* i. 19. 12 quote
nicely from Rose Macaulay, *Staying with Relations*, p. 19
'Squealings and tramplings came from the forest on the left.
Isie said, "Plenty of pig in there." And Catherine surmised,
from her use of the singular number, that she would fain pursue
these animals and take their lives.'

**51. non . . . iubebo :** 'I am not going to tell you . . .' Though
softened by a negative, 'iubebo' is in the most formal didactic
manner; cf. *Georgics* iii. 329–30 'ad puteos aut alta greges ad
stagna iubebo / currentem ilignis potare canalibus undam.'

**53–4.** The subjunctives 'portarit' and 'rapta sit' are concessive—
'I know Perseus brought back Andromeda from Ethiopia, and
Paris had to go to Greece for his girl.'

**53. nigris . . . ab Indis :** In fact Andromeda came from Ethiopia.
The trouble starts with Homer, who divided the Ethiopians
into two groups, eastern and western (*Od.* i. 23–4), and Posi-
donius identified Homer's eastern Ethiopians with the Indians.
Particularly in Latin poetry 'Indians' and 'Ethiopians' are
more or less interchangeable (see J. Y. Nadeau, *CQ* N.S. 20
(1970), 339–49). 'Nigris' may allude to the etymology of Αἰθίωψ
as 'burnt face'.

**56. 'haec habet' ut dicas 'quicquid in orbe fuit'**; cf. Propertius iii.
22. 17–18 'omnia Romanae cedent miracula terrae; / Natura hic
posuit quicquid ubique fuit.' We have here a most ingenious
and amusing parody of a stock patriotic theme of the day—
panegyric of Rome and Italy. Further examples are Varro, *de
Re Rustica* i. 2. 3 ff., Virgil, *Georgics* ii. 136 ff., and later Pliny,
*N.H.* iii. 40–2 and xxxvii. 201. Such passages regularly in-
sist on the all-round excellence and variety of native Italian
products (e.g. Varro, loc. cit. 'quid in Italia utensile non modo
non nascitur, sed etiam non egregium fit?') which made few
imports from abroad necessary. Listen to the contemporary
Dionysius of Halicarnassus praising Italy (*Ant. Rom.* i. 36): 'I
judge supreme the country which is most self-sufficient, and
least in need of imported goods. And I am convinced that Italy
more than any other land possesses this quality of producing
and providing everything.' The same, says Ovid, is true of girls.

57. **Gargara quot segetes :** in the Troad—Gargarus was the highest summit of the range of Ida, and also a town at the mountain's foot. For its harvests, cf. *Georgics* i. 103 'ipsa suas mirantur Gargara messes.'

   **Methymna :** a town on Lesbos, noted for fine vintages (e.g. Prop. iv. 8. 38).

58. **aequore quot pisces :** understand 'teguntur' from the next clause.

59. **quot caelum stellas, tot habet tua Roma puellas :** a pleasant line, made memorable by the rhyme 'stellas . . . puellas', which is perhaps more characteristic of medieval Latin poetry. It seems that in reading aloud the normal spoken stress on the penultimate of a disyllabic word (stéllas) would prevail over the metrical ictus (stellás) ; see W. S. Allen, *Vox Latina* (1965), 92–4.

   A comparison with the stars in the sky for number is of course very common. But Ovid may have in mind a closely parallel passage of Herodas, according to whom Ptolemaic Alexandria in the middle of the third century B.C. contained γυναῖκες ὁκόσους οὐ μὰ τὴν Ἅιδεω Κούρην / ἀστέρας ἐνεγκεῖν οὐρανὸς κεκαύχηται (i. 32–3, 'women in greater numbers, by Persephone, than the sky can boast stars').

60. **mater in Aeneae constitit urbe sui :** cf. *Amores* i. 8. 41–2 'nunc Mars externis animos exercet in armis, / at Venus Aeneae regnat in urbe sui.' Tracing back the *gens Iulia* to Iulus, son of Aeneas, had political advantages, brilliantly exploited by Virgil. But to a lively wit like Ovid's it provided some irreverent associations. For example, Cupid could be reckoned a distant cousin of the emperor—'aspice cognati felicia Caesaris arma' (*Amores* i. 2. 51).

   **constitit :** 'has settled' (cf. Propertius iii. 18. 8 'quis deus in uestra constitit hostis aqua?'), with a suggestion of alighting from heavenly regions (*Aeneid* iv. 252–3 'hic primum paribus nitens Cyllenius alis / constitit').

63. **iuuenem :** of course a young *woman* in her prime, cf. Pliny, *N.H.* vii. 122 'Cornelia . . . iuuenis est et parere adhuc potest.'

64. 'You will be at a loss which one to desire.'

67–262. *Where to find your girl.* Ovid surveys the favourite meeting-places both in Rome and further afield. Lines 67–88 are particularly interesting to us; most of these splendid buildings had been newly erected by Augustus, and we get a vivid impression of the capital city with its temples, colonnades, and fountains. Touches like 'externo marmore' (70) and 'facto de marmore templo' (81) recall the emperor's boast (Suetonius, *Div. Aug.* 28. 2) 'marmoream [sc. urbem] se relinquere quam latericiam accepisset'; whether he would approve of his great works being recommended for assignations is another matter.

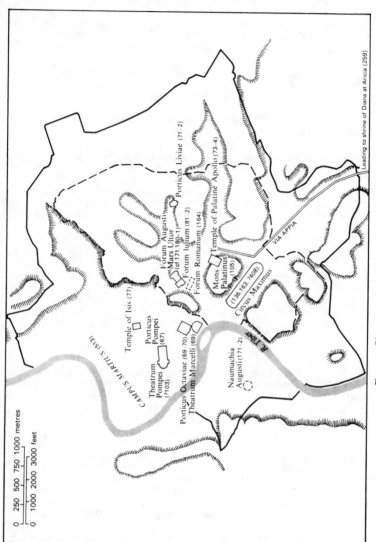

Roman Sites mentioned in *Ars Amatoria* I

(Numbers in brackets denote lines of passages where the sites are mentioned)

I have marked the Ovidian sites on the sketch-map (p. 44). Readers may like to follow the text further with Platner and Ashby, *A Topographical Dictionary of Ancient Rome* (Oxford, 1929), whose work is brought up to date together with magnificent photographs by Ernest Nash, *Pictorial Dictionary of Ancient Rome* (2 vols., London, 1961 and 1962). Corresponding to this passage, girls receive advice where to meet young men at iii. 387 ff.

To gain attractiveness from lively topographical details was a traditional device, possibly originating in Greek New Comedy; compare Plautus, *Amphitruo* 1011 ff., *Curculio* 467 ff. (note 472–3 'dites, damnosos maritos sub basilica quaerito. / ibidem erunt scorta exoleta quique stipulari solent'), Catullus 55.

**67–8.** *You need only stroll along Pompey's Colonnade during the hottest period of the year.* Pompey built his *porticus* in 55 B.C. at the same time as the theatre, to provide shelter for spectators in case of rain. It was a rectangular court about 180 metres long and 135 wide, in which there were four parallel rows of columns. The central area was laid out as a garden with shady walks. At once it became a resort for elegant females (Catullus 55. 6–7 'in Magni simul ambulatione / femellas omnes, amice, prendi'). Propertius (ii. 32. 11–12) paints a luxurious picture, 'umbrosis . . . Pompeia columnis / porticus, aulaeis nobilis Attalicis'.

**67. tu modo Pompeia lentus spatiare sub umbra :** an echo of Propertius iv. 8. 75 (Cynthia laying down the law to her lover) 'tu neque Pompeia spatiabere cultus in umbra.' Both 'lentus' and 'spatiare' suggest a leisured stroll, allowing plenty of time to observe the surroundings. Ovid in turn was imitated by Martial xi. 47. 3 'cur nec Pompeia lentus spatiatur in umbra?'

**68.** The sun enters the zodiacal sign Leo on approximately 23 July, so this is the hottest time of the year, when the shady walks would provide welcome relief.

**Herculei . . . leonis :** because the constellation Leo was supposed to represent the Nemean lion (killed by Hercules) raised to the skies.

**69–70. aut ubi muneribus nati sua munera mater / addidit :** He refers to the Porticus of Octavia (the mother) and the adjoining Theatre of Marcellus (her son). The *Porticus Octaviae* (not to be confused with the *Porticus Octavia* of 168 B.C., restored by Octavian in 33 B.C.) was dedicated in the name of the emperor's sister some time after 27 B.C.; see Nash, *Pictorial Dictionary*, vol. II, figs. 1004–8. Construction of the *Theatrum Marcelli* (Nash, vol. II, figs. 1210–15) was so advanced in 17 B.C. that parts of the *ludi saeculares* could be celebrated within the theatre, but the dedication did not occur until (probably) 13 B.C. One would naturally deduce from Ovid's words that the

*Porticus Octaviae* followed the *Theatrum Marcelli*, but he might be speaking just of a library in the porticus specifically commemorating Octavia's son Marcellus who died in 23 B.C. (Plutarch, *Marcellus* 30. 6).

**70. externo marmore :** foreign marble. On the importing of marble, see A. Boethius and J. B. Ward-Perkins, *Etruscan and Roman Architecture* (1970), pp. 116, 260 ff. Probably we should imagine coloured foreign marble setting off the brilliant white of the Italian Carrara stone (cf. ibid., p. 191 on the *Forum Augustum*).

**71–2.** The *Porticus Liviae*, built on the site of Vedius Pollio's house (for whom see Dio liv. 23), was dedicated to the empress Livia in 7 B.C. No other authority seems to mention its pictures ('priscis . . . tabellis', 71), but e.g. the *Porticus Pompei* and the *Porticus Octaviae* (above) contained many notable works of art (references in Platner and Ashby).

**73–4.** Most magnificent of all Augustus' works, the temple of Palatine Apollo was vowed in 36 B.C. during the campaign against Sextus Pompey, begun the same year and dedicated on 9 October 28 B.C. Propertius (ii. 31) gives us a conducted tour; see also Nisbet and Hubbard on Horace, *Odes* i. 31. 1. Identifying any remains has proved a problem (cf. Nash, *Pictorial Dictionary*, figs. 23–4).

The temple was connected with, and perhaps surrounded by, a porticus between the columns of which stood statues of the fifty daughters of Danaus (*Belides*, 74, also mentioned in *Tristia* iii. 1. 61–2, Prop. ii. 31. 4) and, presumably, of Danaus himself (*pater*, 74). For female company in these surroundings cf. *Amores* ii. 2. 3–4 'hesterna uidi spatiantem luce puellam / illa quae Danai porticus agmen habet.'

**74. Belides :** so called after their grandfather Belus, who was father to Danaus and Aegyptus. The fifty sons of Aegyptus pursued the fifty daughters of Danaus from Egypt to Greece, and gained their hand in marriage. But on the wedding night all except one (Hypermestra) of the Danaids murdered their cousin-husbands (cf. 73 *patruelibus*). Ovid clearly represents Danaus as egging his daughters on. This legend was the subject of a trilogy by Aeschylus, from which we have only the first play, *Supplices*.

**75–6.** We switch briefly to occasions rather than places (77–8 return to places, but are linked to 75–6 by the religious theme). That the hero should meet the heroine at a religious festival was a favourite literary motif, above all in New Comedy (see Headlam on Herodas 1. 56, Gow on Theocritus 2. 66 ff.). It had a basis of fact, because in Greece festivals were among the few occasions when a respectable young woman might be seen in public.

**75.** On the festival of the *Adonia*, see Gow's introduction to Theo-
critus, *Id.* 15 (vol. II, pp. 262–4). Some lines of the New Comedy
poet Diphilus (fr. 43. 39–40 Edmonds, *ap.* Athenaeus vii. 292d)
suggest that the *Adonia* was observed particularly by *hetaerae*;
cf. also Dioscorides, *Anth. Pal.* v. 193.

   **nec te praetereat :** not Lucretian or Virgilian, but in Manilius
(e.g. ii. 203). Compare in Greek didactic verse e.g. Aratus 607–8
οὐδ' ἂν ἐπερχόμεναι Χηλαί . . . / ἄφραστοι παρίοιεν, Nicander, *Theriaca*
583 μηδὲ σέ . . . λάθοι.

**76.** **cultaque Iudaeo septima sacra Syro :** an interesting indication
(see also 415–16) of how far Judaism had affected Rome's social
and economic life. G. La Piana (*Harvard Theological Review* 20
(1927), 352 ff.) records no fewer than thirteen Roman syna-
gogues. Attached to these would be believing Gentiles ('God-
fearers', *metuentes*, οἱ σεβόμενοι τὸν θεόν, cf. Jean Juster, *Les Juifs
dans l'Empire romain* (Paris, 1914), pp. 274 ff.), a high proportion
of them women, who yet did not observe the full rigour of the
Jewish law. No doubt their knowledge and commitment varied
widely, stretching down to idle curiosity which made them con-
gregate outside the synagogue on a Sabbath.

   After the capture of Jerusalem by Pompey in 63 B.C. many
Jews came to Rome as prisoners of war, later gaining their
liberty and staying in the capital (cf. Philo, *Legatio ad Gaium*
155). Julius Caesar showed them great favour, and Augustus
continued the same benevolent policy. It may be that the
position of synagogues in Rome was officially confirmed in 7 B.C.
(Smallwood on Philo, *Legatio ad Gaium* 156). Juster (op. cit.,
p. 209) estimates the size of the colony during Tiberius' reign at
between 50,000 and 60,000; over 8,000 Roman Jews accompanied
an embassy from Palestine to the emperor in A.D. 4 (Josephus,
*A.J.* xvii. 300, *B.J.* ii. 80). Prominent Romans were struck by
the Jews' imageless worship (Varro *ap.* Augustine, *de Civ. Dei*
iv. 31. 2), their observance of the Sabbath (a letter of Augustus
to Tiberius *ap.* Suetonius, *Div. Aug.* 76. 2) and proselytizing
zeal (Horace, *Sat.* i. 4. 143). Harry J. Leon, *The Jews of Ancient
Rome* (1960), ch. 1, discusses many of these Gentile comments
interestingly. The Jewish religion also probably helped to
establish a seven-day week in Rome (Balsdon, *Life and Leisure
in Ancient Rome*, p. 62).

**77–8.** **nec fuge linigerae Memphitica templa iuuencae / (multas
illa facit, quod fuit ipsa Ioui) :** This couplet depends on identi-
fication of Isis with the Greek heroine Io, daughter of Inachus;
she was once the mistress of Zeus and now gets many other
women into the same position (for Io's story cf. e.g. *Met.* i.
583 ff.). Herodotus (ii. 59) had equated Isis with Demeter, but he
recognized (ii. 41) that Isis and Io had similar iconography, both

being represented in human shape but with horns. The identifi-
cation with Io was established by the time of Callimachus (*Ep.*
57. I *Ἰναχίης . . . Ἰσιδος*).

Concerning the unsavoury reputation of Isis in Rome cf.
Juvenal 9. 22 ff., Martial xi. 47. 4; the main temple was in the
Campus Martius. This cult did not fare so well as Judaism at the
hands of the authorities, and we hear of measures against it
under both Augustus and Tiberius. But undoubtedly it remained
popular, particularly with women—the heroines of Roman elegy
are regularly portrayed as devotees of Isis.

77. **linigerae :** The priests of Isis wore linen clothes, avoiding wool,
which they considered an impure excrement (cf. Herodotus ii.
37 and 81, Plutarch, *Isis and Osiris* 4).

**Memphitica :** hardly more then 'Egyptian'. But there might
be an allusion to the temple of Isis which the Pharaoh Amasis
built in the sixth century B.C. at Memphis (Herodotus ii.176).

**79–88.** *Believe it or not, a love affair can even start in the law courts.*

79. **et fora :** 'even *fora*'.

**(quis credere possit?):** One would not imagine that long-winded
treatises and turgid rhetoric left much room for intimate emo-
tions. Unlike his brother, Ovid was temperamentally ill-suited
to the law (*Tristia* iv. 10. 17 ff.) and states his dislike of the pro-
fession (*Amores* i. 15. 5–6 'nec me uerbosas leges ediscere nec
me / ingrato uocem prostituisse foro'). Even so he had con-
siderable knowledge of legal terminology, and delights to poke
fun at it (see on 83–6 and 585–8). E. J. Kenney, 'Ovid and the
Law' (*Yale Classical Studies* 21 (1969), 243–63) examines the
poet's own career. One should add that rejection of bombastic
oratory was a traditional pose among elegists who practised
Callimachean restraint, as Apollo forbade Propertius 'insano
uerba tonare foro' (iv. I. 134).

80. **in arguto . . . foro :** changing from plural to singular because
he already begins to particularize, referring to the *Forum
Iulium* (see on 81–2). For this reason I prefer no punctuation
after 80, but a colon after 82. This also provides a better
structure for the whole passage, continuing the sequence of
four-line units (67–70, 71–4, 75–8, 79–82, 83–6).

**arguto :** clearly in a bad sense, 'shrill', 'wordy'.

81–8. Paul Turner's translation sparkles, matching point for
point—inevitably not quite the same point as in Ovid (see on
83–6): 'You know where the Appian fountain spurts into the
air, just below the temple of Venus? Well, that is where many
a learned friend has been transformed into a lover, and many
a legal adviser has acted most ill-advisedly. There the fluent
speaker is always liable to dry up, as a fresh piece of evidence

suddenly catches his eye, and he finds he will have to plead his
own cause. From her marble home next door Venus laughs to
see a barrister so badly in need of Counsel.'

**81–2. subdita qua Veneris facto de marmore templo / Appias
expressis aera pulsat aquis :** We are in the *Forum Iulium*, where
stands the fountain of the Appiades. Behind the fountain steps
lead up to the temple of Venus Genetrix. The scene is portrayed
on a coin of Trajan, illustrated by Nash (*Pictorial Dictionary*,
vol. I fig. 26, whence my Plate I) who also photographed the site
as it is now (fig. 25), showing what may be the foundation walls
of the Appiades. Julius Caesar dedicated the *Forum Iulium* and
temple of Venus Genetrix in 46 B.C., although both works had
subsequently to be completed by Augustus (see Nash, vol. I
figs. 519–29). Caesar planned his forum not as a market, but for
other kinds of business (Appian, *B.C.* ii. 102), and, appropriately
enough, Ovid shows us the lawyers practising there.

**82. Appias :** the fountain's water-nymph (cf. *Remedia* 660). But
the reason for this name eludes us, since the *Aqua Appia* did not
extend to that part of Rome. At iii. 452 Ovid speaks of Appiades
in the plural, and Asinius Pollio's art collection boasted an
'Appiades' by Stephanus (Pliny, *N.H.* xxxvi. 33), perhaps a
copy of the work in the *Forum Iulium*. So there may have been
more than one figure of a nymph.

   **expressis aera pulsat aquis :** A jet of water spurts out under
high pressure, possibly from the mouth of the nymph. Roman
ornamental fountains then as now might be highly ingenious;
cf. Clemens Herschel, *Frontinus and the Water Supply of the
City of Rome* (1899), ch. 8, and e.g. Propertius ii. 32. 13–16.

**83–6.** Every line contains a double meaning based on legal ter-
minology—a notable tour de force.

**83. capitur :** 'is trapped'. Under the obvious amatory sense (e.g.
61, Propertius i. 1. 1) there lies a technical lawyer's use of *capi*,
meaning to be tricked by a form of words. It would of course be
the business of a *iurisconsultus* to ensure that his client did not
suffer this fate: 'tu caues ne tui consultores . . . capiantur'
(Cicero, *pro Murena* 22). Compare the formula at Cicero, *de
Officiis* iii. 70 'uti ne propter te fidemue tuam captus fraudatusue
sim' (see further Douglas on Cic., *Brutus* 178).

   **consultus :** the legal expert (*iure-* or *iurisconsultus*) as opposed
to the forensic orator (*disertus*) in 85. For this division cf.
*Amores* i. 13. 21 'nec tu consulto nec tu iucunda diserto', Cicero,
*Brutus* 148 'consultorum alterum disertissimum, disertorum
alterum consultissimum'.

   **Amori :** dative of the agent after a passive verb, cf. Horace,
*Epist.* i. 19. 3 'quae scribuntur aquae potoribus'.

**84. quique aliis cauit, non cauet ipse sibi :** The first use of *cauere* is

rigidly technical of a *iurisconsultus* = pro clientibus cautionum
(a bond or pledge to secure the position of one party) formulas
scribere (*T.L.L.* s.v. *caueo* III A), the second more general = to
look out for oneself. Cicero teases his jurist friend Trebatius in
exactly the same way: 'tu qui ceteris *cauere* didicisti, in Britan-
nia ne ab essedariis decipiaris *caueto*' (*ad Fam.* vii. 6. 2). There
were also plenty of ancient proverbs about e.g. philosophers or
doctors who could not apply their skill to themselves; see Otto,
*Sprichwörter* s.v. *sapere*, Phaedrus i. 9. 1–2 'sibi non cauere et
aliis consilium dare / stultum esse paucis ostendamus uersibus.'

**85. desunt sua uerba diserto :** 'the barrister's words abandon him'
(for *disertus* as a substantive see on 83). Below the surface mean-
ing (e.g. Plautus, *Bacchides* 37 'ne defuerit mihi in monendo
oratio') lurks another image—that of an influential citizen
failing to help a friend or client by speaking in court of his good
character. Compare Cicero, *pro Sex. Roscio* 30 'patronos huic
defuturos putaverunt; desunt.'

**86. res . . . nouae :** a case for which there is no precedent (*Vocabu-
larium Iurisprudentiae Romanae*, vol. V col. 107 s.v. *res noua*).
The barrister's professional experience cannot help him when he
first falls in love; he has never met this situation before.

**87. hunc Venus . . . ridet :** the Homeric 'laughter-loving Aphrodite'
(φιλομμείδης Ἀφροδίτη, 'Erycina ridens' in Horace, *Odes* i. 2. 33).
Her smile became fixed in later poetry; cf. Sappho, *Lyrica
Graeca Selecta* (Page) 191. 14 μειδιαίσαισ' ἀθανάτῳ προσώπῳ, Theo-
critus 1. 94 ἦνθέ γε μὰν ἁδεῖα καὶ ἁ Κύπρις γελάοισα, Horace, *Odes* ii. 8.
13 'ridet hoc, inquam, Venus.'

    **templis :** the temple of Venus Genetrix (see on 81–2).

**89–134.** *But your best hunting-ground is the theatre. This has been so
ever since the time of Romulus* (101–34, interlude on the Rape of
the Sabine Women).

**90. uoto . . . tuo :** ablative of comparison, 'even more productive
than you could wish'.

**91–2. quod ames, quod ludere possis, / quodque semel tangas,
quodque tenere uelis :** for the neuter cf. 35 n. Ovid effectively
divides the women into two classes with chiasmus—'a girl to
love, a girl to deceive, a girl to leave, a girl to keep' (Kenney).

**91. ludere :** 'to deceive', as at 643. With an accusative (*quod*) the
verb can hardly mean 'to flirt with'; we would expect *cum* or *in*
+ablative.

**93–6.** Both these comparisons recall Virgil—the ants *Aeneid* iv.
402–7 and the bees *Georgics* iv. 162–9 (repeated almost word for
word at *Aeneid* i. 430–6). They illustrate different aspects of the
scene. The ants call to mind an unbroken column making
purposefully for the theatre (cf. *Aen.* iv. 405 'calle angusto',

Aristotle, *Historia Animalium* ix. 38. 622b 'they all continually travel on a single path', Ovid line 93 'longum . . . per agmen') while the bees add a touch of elegance and perhaps imply that the girls' attention is easily turned from one sight to another (cf. 96).

**93. redit itque :** the natural order reversed for metrical reasons (see Kenney on Lucretius iii. 787).

**agmen :** cf. *Aen.* iv. 404 'it nigrum campis agmen.' Servius supplies the curious information that the same words had been used twice before—by Ennius of elephants and by Accius of Indians. But why does Ovid write '*per* agmen'? It seems almost that he imagined the column as existing independently of the ants which form it, so that they can be said to move *along* the column.

**94. granifero :** cf. *Met.* vii. 638 (also of ants). The compound does not survive elsewhere.

**95–6.** The simile is redolent of Virgil's *Georgics* (but note that crowding women are likened to bees earlier in Ap. Rh. i. 879 ff.). Compare particularly iv. 54–6 'illae (the bees) continuo saltus siluasque peragrant, / purpureosque metunt flores et flumina libant / summa leues', and for 'nactae' iv. 77. Virgil himself fashioned iv. 162–9 into a simile at *Aen.* i. 430–6.

**99. spectatum ueniunt, ueniunt spectentur ut ipsae :** an ingenious line. Perhaps remembering Plautus, *Poenulus* 337 'sunt illi aliae quas spectare ego et me spectari volo', Ovid turns to his advantage an argument which had been used against such displays. One can cite a remark supposedly addressed by Socrates to Xanthippe, 'You see, you are not going for the spectacle, but rather to make a spectacle of yourself' (Aelian, *Var. Hist.* vii. 10). Christian writers made the same point in their condemnation of Games, e.g. Tertullian, *de Spectaculis* 25 'nemo denique in spectaculo ineundo prius cogitat nisi uidere et uideri.'

**101–34.** Interlude, *The Rape of the Sabine Women*. Ovid presents this in the learned Hellenistic manner as an aetiological tale— ever since then the theatre has been a dangerous place for pretty girls (see on 133–4 for the formal conclusion). It is one of his most pleasant creations. We must imagine the mixed reactions of a Roman audience. The Augustans were particularly fond of stories of their city's infancy, and the Rape of the Sabine Women was firmly established in tradition (cf. R. M. Ogilvie on Livy i. 9, also Dionysius Hal., *Ant. Rom.* ii. 30, Plutarch, *Romulus* 14). But obviously it must have embarrassed upholders of Roman *gravitas*. The women themselves became proverbial for chastity (Juvenal 6. 163–4 'intactior omni / crinibus effusis bellum dirimente Sabina'), though one might view them otherwise. Ovid pokes fun at the primitive character of early Rome (see on 103 ff.), and enthusiastically applauds Romulus' action (131–2), claiming in effect that the Founder had anticipated his own doctrines (101)! To crown the whole piece, lines 131–2 cast a sly glance at contemporary recruiting difficulties in the Roman army.

A. E. Wardman (*CQ* N.S. 15 (1965), 101–3) points out that the action was normally placed at chariot-races in the Circus. Although preserving a trace of this version (105–6 n.) Ovid transfers the scene to the theatre. Thereby he mocks (a) censorious criticism of the theatre (cf. particularly Tacitus, *Annals* xiv. 20) by suggesting that lax behaviour there, far from being a foreign importation, had existed from Rome's earliest days, and (b) the segregation of the sexes (109 n.)—if Romulus could organize the affair in a segregated theatre, his descendants can hardly be blamed for more sophisticated adventures.

**101. primus sollicitos fecisti, Romule, ludos :** perhaps an echo of Propertius on the *spolia opima*, 'imbuis exemplum primae tu, Romule, palmae / huius' (iv. 10. 5–6). Ovid here parodies the ancient preoccupation with inventors. Since the time of Aristotle scholars had written works περὶ εὑρημάτων, ascribing each innovation to a named individual (see Nisbet and Hubbard on Horace, *Odes* i. 3. 12, and my note on *Met.* viii. 244–5). In didactic poetry too inventors came to have an established place; the author will call down blessings on the man who made a notable advance in technique, as does Ovid in 131–2 and Grattius in *Cynegetica* i. 95 ff., 215–16 'Hagnon, quem plurima semper / gratia per nostros unum testabitur usus'. Virgil's *Georgics* offer Aristaeus as inventor of βουγονία (iv. 315–16), Ericthonius of the four-horse chariot and the Lapiths of the bridle (iii. 113–17). Note also the beginning of [Oppian], *Cyn.* ii.

**102. uiduos :** 'wifeless'—they were not of course widowers! Compare Livy i. 9. 1 'penuria mulierum hominis aetatem duratura magnitudo erat, quippe quibus nec domi spes prolis nec cum finitimis conubia essent.'

**103 ff.** Romans of the Augustan age delighted to picture the primitive state of their city. They liked to ask with Propertius (iv. 4. 9) 'quid tum Roma fuit?'; mingled with pride in what the city had become there was nostalgia for the time when sheep had grazed on the site of all those splendid buildings. We have many passages which gain their effect by making a sharp contrast between present magnificence and past simplicity. Thus Propertius iv. 1. 1 ff.:

> Hoc quodcunque uides, hospes, qua maxima Roma est,
>     ante Phrygem Aenean collis et herba fuit;
> atque ubi Nauali stant sacra Palatia Phoebo,
>     Euandri profugae procubuere boues *etc.*

and, viewed from the other end, Virgil on Aeneas' visit to
Evander at the site of future Rome (*Aen.* viii. 360–1):

> passimque armenta uidebant
> Romanoque foro et lautis mugire Carinis.

Compare further Tibullus ii. 5. 23 ff., Prop. iv. 4. 9 ff., and in less
idyllic manner Martial i. 2, Juvenal 3. 12 ff.

Ovid writes in the same tradition, but his attitude to the past
is far from reverential. He amuses himself over the crude
entertainment (103–7, 111–13), the men's uncouth appearance
and primitive sunshades (108), and the careful way in which
they stare at the Sabine women, each marking out one for him-
self and silently brooding over his plans (109–10).

**103–4.** Compare Propertius iv. 1. 15–16 (also on primitive Rome)
'nec sinuosa cauo pendebant uela theatro, / pulpita solemnes
non oluere crocos.'

**103. tunc neque marmoreo pendebant uela theatro :** He is prob-
ably thinking of the *Theatrum Pompei* (which was in fact some-
times called 'theatrum marmoreum'), built in 55 B.C., Rome's
first permanent theatre and always the most important. See
Nash, *Pictorial Dictionary*, figs. 1216–23; fig. 1217 shows
remarkably how the outline of modern buildings preserves the
plan of the theatre. As for the awnings (*uela*) stretched over the
top, Q. Lutatius Catulus introduced this idea at the dedication
of the Capitoline temple (see Pliny, *N.H.* xix. 23). The awnings
would be supported on transverse beams slung between up-
right masts; holes for such masts have been found in the
Colosseum (see Boethius and Ward-Perkins, *Etruscan and
Roman Architecture*, p. 224). Lucretius uses the gaily-coloured
awnings for one of his most notable illustrations from Roman
life (iv. 75 ff.). It is worth quoting the first three lines:

> et uulgo faciunt id lutea russaque uela
> et ferrugina, cum magnis intenta theatris
> per malos uulgata trabesque trementia flutant.

**104. nec fuerant liquido pulpita rubra croco :** Pounded saffron
would be mixed with sweet wine, and sprayed on to the stage, to
produce a pleasant perfume (Pliny, *N.H.* xxi. 33). Besides
Propertius iv. 1. 16 (above) cf. Lucretius ii. 416 'cum scaena
croco Cilici perfusa recens est'.

**105–6.** The incident took place in the Vallis Murcia, lying between
the Palatine and Aventine hills, site of the future Circus Maxi-
mus. Its occasion was the Consualia, a festival in honour of
Consus (generally held to have been god of Consilium—cf.
Tertullian quoted on 133–4—though a link with *condere* is more
probable).

**105. Palatia :** according to all ancient traditions the first of the seven hills to be occupied.

**106. scena sine arte fuit :** the phrase with *sine* functions as a Greek adjective with α- privative. Ovid himself would have been familiar with elaborate stage scenery (cf. Val. Max. ii. 4. 6, W. Beare, *The Roman Stage*, Appendix H, Margarete Bieber, *The History of the Greek and Roman Theater*, chs. 13–15 (copiously illustrated). But here there are only boughs piled up behind the players.

**107. gradibus . . . de caespite factis :** They sit on the lower slopes of the Palatine to get a better view. 'Factis' does not imply any special preparation of the seats; rather it points a contrast with the wooden or stone seats of later days.

**108.** The rape was thought to have occurred in high summer (18 August, the festival of the Consualia), so they break off a leafy branch to act as a sunshade. These branches correspond to the *uela* of the poet's time (103).

  **hirsutas . . . comas :** not having the benefit of Ovid's advice on hair-style (517–18).

**109–10.** Livy (i. 9. 11) imagines that it was pure chance which girl each man ended up with: 'magna pars forte in quem quaeque inciderat raptae' (cf. Dion. Hal., *Ant. Rom.* ii. 30. 4 'whichever one they chanced upon'). But here at least Ovid makes the Romans act more scientifically, in accordance with his own precept 'quaerenda est oculis apta puella tuis' (44).

**109. respiciunt :** Seating arrangements are as in Augustan Rome. The emperor laid down that women should occupy only the back rows in the theatre (Suetonius, *Div. Aug.* 44); cf. *Amores* ii. 7. 3 'siue ego marmorei respexi summa theatri', Propertius iv. 8. 77.

**110. multa mouent :** an epic phrase (*Aeneid* v. 608), sometimes with *animo* added (*Aen.* iii. 34, x. 890). For 'tacito pectore' cf. also *Aen.* i. 502.

**111–12.** The entertainment consists of dancing to a musical accompaniment, in the Etruscan manner. According to Livy (vii. 2) this was first introduced in 364–3 B.C. as part of the remedies for a plague: 'ludiones ex Etruria acciti, ad tibicinis modos saltantes, haud indecoros motus more Tusco dabant.' For a discussion of Livy, see W. Beare, *The Roman Stage*, pp. 16–23.

**112. aequatam ter pede pulsat humum :** cf. Horace, *Odes* iii. 18. 15–16 'gaudet inuisam pepulisse fossor / ter pede terram.'

  **aequatam . . . humum :** equivalent to the *pulpita* (104, cf. 108 n.).

  **ter pede :** suggesting 'tripudium', a wild ritual dance particularly associated with the Salii or 'leaping' priests, for whom see Ogilvie on Livy i. 20. 3–4. The implied etymology may well be sound, in spite of Cicero, *de Divinatione* ii. 72. Beare (*The Roman Stage*, p. 16) tentatively connects the tripudium with Saturnian rhythm.

**pulsat** : a vigorous and inelegant motion (cf. Horace, *Odes* i. 37. 1–2 'nunc pede libero / pulsanda tellus')—even though Ennius wrote of the Muses 'Musae quae pedibus magnum pulsatis Olympum' (*Annals* 1 Warmington). For the uninhibited character of old Roman dancing cf. Seneca, *de Tranquillitate Animi* 17 'Scipio triumphale illud ac militare corpus mouebat ad numeros . . . ut antiqui illi uiri solebant inter lusum ac festa tempora uirilem in modum tripudiare.'

**113. (plausus tunc arte carebant):** in contrast to the organised rhythmical applause which reached its height when the emperor Nero performed. Suetonius (*Nero* 20) even speaks of 'plausuum genera . . . bombos et imbrices et testas'; cf. Tacitus, *Annals* xvi. 5.

**114. praedae signa †petenda† :** For discussion of the text see Kenney, *CQ* N.S. 9 (1959), 242–3 and Goold, *Harvard Studies* 69 (1965), 60–1. 'Petenda' can hardly stand. To take the phrase as = 'signa praedae petendae' would put an intolerable strain on the Latin, while translation as 'the signal to be awaited' misrepresents *peto*; the meaning should be 'the signal which they had to demand', but this is an absurdity (Kenney). The most probable emendation, due to Bentley and Madvig, is 'petita', 'the signal they had been looking for' (Goold). One need not worry about praeda = the *act* of plundering (praedatio); see R. G. Nisbet on Cicero, *de Domo* 50.

Among other tries Josef Delz (*Museum Helveticum* 28 (1971), 52–3) would revive Burman's 'repente', a word not common in poetry but occupying the same position at *Tristia* iii. 8. 8—it seems, however, to lack sharpness after 'in medio plausu'— while Kenney (loc. cit.) tentatively proposed 'rex populo praed*am* signa pet*ente* [so alternatively Burman] dedit.'

**117–18.** The comparisons with doves fleeing from eagles (cf. *Iliad* xxii. 139–40) and lambs from a wolf (cf. Theocritus 11. 24) are very conventional; both appear at *Met.* i. 505–6 of an amorous pursuit. Yet we are surprised to learn that in fact some of the Sabine women stay put (122–4).

**118. utque fugit uisos . . . lupos :** One glimpse of a wolf is enough to set the lamb off; cf. Theocritus 11. 24 φεύγεις δ' ὥσπερ ὄις πολιὸν λύκον ἀθρήσασα, Horace, *Odes* i. 15. 29–30 'ceruus uti uallis in altera / uisum parte lupum'. The second parallel can vindicate the text as against 'ut fugit inuisos' (ς) preferred by Goold, op. cit., p. 61 (although his account of the alleged corruption is plausible).

**agna nouella :** The diminutive is not sentimental but agricultural, as e.g. Pliny, *N.H.* xi. 211 'nouellarum suum'.

**121–4.** One may suspect, as often, that Ovid has in mind some pictorial representation. The Romans have leapt up and are making for the Sabine women, while the latter are caught in a great variety of attitudes. Ovid achieves clarity and sharpness of visual detail, combined with the utmost economy of words.

**121. facies non una timoris :** cf. Virgil, *Georgics* i. 506 'tam multae scelerum facies', *Aen.* ii. 369 'plurima mortis imago'.

**122. sedet :** with the implication of sitting dumbly and hopelessly.

**125. ducuntur raptae, genialis praeda, puellae :** For the artificial word order with adjective and noun enclosing a phrase in apposition, see my note on *Met.* viii. 226.

    **genialis praeda :** 'spoil for the marriage bed' (cf. lectus genialis). Appearances notwithstanding, it all turns out to be perfectly proper, as in Livy i. 9. 14 'illas tamen in matrimonio, in societate fortunarum omnium ciuitatisque et, quo nihil carius humano generi sit, liberum fore'.

**126. potuit :** 'it could be that . . .' We are faced with a difficult choice at the end of the line between 'timor' and 'pudor'. The former, which has rather better manuscript support, finds many parallels (e.g. *Met.* iv. 230 'ipse timor decuit', *Fasti* v. 608) and has pleased modern editors. But have we not heard enough about *timor* (119, 121)? The idea that a maidenly blush makes a girl more attractive is equally a commonplace (e.g. *Am.* i. 8. 35 'decet alba quidem pudor ora', Curtius vi. 3. 6 'formam pudor honestabat') and provides a nicer link with 127.

    The reading of S$_a$ 'et patuit multis tunc timor ipse dei' looks like a Christian interpolation; the same may be true of 'deo' for 'Syro' in O at 76 and 416.

**127. si qua repugnarat nimium :** a notion which recurs time and time again in the love-poets. It was right and proper for the girls to put up a show of reluctance, but not to carry their opposition too far (e.g. 665–6, *Amores* i. 5. 13–16, Horace, *Odes* i. 9. 21–4).

    **comitemque negarat :** cf. Horace, *Odes* i. 35. 22 'nec comitem abnegat', with Nisbet and Hubbard ad loc.

**128. sublatam cupido uir tulit ipse sinu :** From this incident antiquarians derive the Roman custom for a husband to carry his bride across the threshold of their new home (see Plutarch, *Romulus* 15)!

**129. 'quid teneros lacrimis corrumpis ocellos?' :** for the verb cf. Plautus, *Amphitruo* 530 'ne corrumpe oculos.' So Catullus complained to Lesbia's dead bird 'tua nunc opera meae puellae / flendo turgiduli rubent ocelli' (3. 17–18).

**130. quod matri pater est, hoc tibi' dixit 'ero.' :** Here again Ovid seems to have one eye on Livy—or at least on traditional justifications of the rape. Compare Livy i. 9. 15 'eoque melioribus usuras uiris quod adnisurus pro se quisque sit ut, cum suam

uicem functus officio sit, parentium etiam patriaeque expleat
desiderium' (see Ogilvie ad loc.).

**131-2. Romule, militibus scisti dare commoda solus : / haec mihi si
dederis commoda, miles ero :** Hans Petersen (*TAPA* 92 (1961),
446) was right to see here a reference to contemporary re-
cruiting difficulties, but he exaggerated in saying that these
lines 'are in themselves perhaps sufficient to explain, if not to
justify, Ovid's exile'.

**131. commoda :** clearly 'fringe benefits', in addition to the
soldiers' regular pay. As a technical term 'commoda' applied
particularly to the retirement gratuity, given either in money or
land; cf. Suetonius, *Div. Aug.* 24 'commoda emeritorum prae-
miorum', *Nero* 32 'stipendia . . . militum et commoda ueterano-
rum' (further examples in the *Thesaurus*). There would also be
distributions of cash to mark special occasions—under later
emperors these became much more important—and in troubled
times soldiers might hope for plunder.

Dio Cassius (lv. 23) expressly states that the lowness of these
extra rewards had been a cause for complaint in the army. In
A.D. 5/6 Augustus was forced to extend the term of service and
to increase payment on discharge; henceforward each legionary
would get 3,000 denarii, perhaps three times the previous amount
(P. A. Brunt 'Pay and Superannuation in the Roman Army',
*B.S.R.* 18 (1950), 50-71, particularly p. 63). So Ovid is saying in
effect, 'If they could offer a pretty girl as a side-attraction
nowadays, that would solve the recruiting problem!'

**solus :** as often, expressing eminence rather than uniqueness
(see Shackleton Bailey on Propertius ii. 34. 26)—'you above all
others', with the clear implication 'you above the present Roman
leader'.

**132.** In spite of the contemporary reference, I doubt whether it is
relevant that Octavian considered taking the name Romulus
rather than Augustus (Dio liii. 16, cf. Suetonius, *Div. Aug.* 7).

**miles ero :** A period of military service was traditional for
Romans of the administrative class, and Augustus had a great
personal concern for this (Suetonius, *Div. Aug.* 38). But,
notoriously, Ovid avoided it; cf. *Amores* i. 15. 3-4 (a complaint
of Jealousy) 'non me more patrum, dum strenua sustinet aetas, /
praemia militiae puluerulenta sequi'.

**133-4. scilicet ex illo sollemni more theatra / nunc quoque formosis
insidiosa manent :** the formal conclusion, linking up with 101.
For the phraseology Kenney compares Ap. Rh. iv. 250-2 τό γε
μὴν ἔδος ἐξέτι κείνου (*ex illo*) / . . . ἀνδράσιν ὀψιγόνοισι μένει καὶ τῆμος (*nunc
quoque . . . manent*) ἰδέσθαι. Learned Hellenistic poets liked to
relate their stories to surviving landmarks, ceremonies etc.;
besides the *Aetia* of Callimachus cf. Phanocles fr. 1. 27-8 Powell,

and my notes on *Met.* viii. 251–9 (the *Ornithogonia* of Boeus) and viii. 719–20 (the *Heteroeumena* of Nicander).

On the more recent reputation of theatres it is interesting to compare Tertullian's biting scorn (*de Spectaculis* 5): 'et Consualia Romulo defendunt, quod ea Conso dicauerit deo, ut uolunt, consilii—eius scilicet quo tunc Sabinarum uirginum rapinam militibus suis excogitauit. probum plane consilium et *nunc quoque inter ipsos Romanos iustum et licitum!*' The italicized words almost suggest that Tertullian had read Ovid and found in him a unexpected ally (see also 99 n.). Propertius too blamed the moral laxity of contemporary Rome on its founder (ii. 6. 19–22):

> tu criminis auctor
> nutritus duro, Romule, lacte lupae.
> tu rapere intactas docuisti impune Sabinas:
> per te nunc Romae quidlibet audet Amor.

**133. scilicet :** in the literal and emphatic sense. Kenney (in *Ovidiana*, p. 202) notes this as a traditional didactic touch, citing Lucretius i. 377, 439 etc., Virgil, *Georgics* ii. 61.

**ex illo :** 'from that time'. Quite apart from the parallel at *Heroides* 14. 85 'scilicet ex illo Iunonia permanet ira' one could hardly take 'ex illo . . . more' together. The rape of the Sabine women was a single act performed once, not a *mos*.

**sollemni more theatra:** For the text see Kenney, *CQ* 1959, 243, and Goold, *Harvard Studies* 69 (1965), 62. Madvig's emendation 'sollemni' for 'sollemnia', 'by hallowed custom' (Goold) is in fact the reading of the *Hamiltonensis* (Y) and would now be accepted by Kenney, who compares Lucretius i. 96–7 'sollemni more sacrorum / perfecto'. Tränkle (*Hermes* 1972, 393 n. 4) adds in support [Virgil], *Ciris* 127, Suetonius *Div. Aug.* 56.

**135–62.** *Finding a girl at the chariot races in the Circus Maximus.*

This section is a great disappointment, and a strong support for those who consider the *Amores* superior to the *Ars Amatoria*. We are offered a pallid reworking of the brilliant and delightful *Amores* iii. 2 (readers will enjoy L. P. Wilkinson's translation, *Ovid Recalled*, pp. 57–60). In both places the situation is the same, and Ovid makes extensive verbal borrowing from his earlier poem. But in recasting the monologue as advice to another he dissipates nearly all the wit. Many themes vanish almost without trace, e.g. the ingenious linking of the poet's success or failure to win the girl with the success or failure of the charioteer whom she supports (only line 146 remains). We miss the delicate hint that Ovid already knows the girl—though not a follower of the Turf he has come to be with her (*Am.* iii. 2. 1–4)

—but only slightly, so that he is tentative and unsure of success. In the *Ars* the prospective lover is meeting a girl for the first time (cf. 144). The running commentary on the race has gone, and so have other delights, e.g. the way Ovid is brought down from the clouds to observe that her feet will not reach the ground and to suggest that she stick her toes into the railings in front (*Am.* iii. 2. 63–4). All that remains is a catalogue of the small offices which one can perform for the girl (149–62). Happily, few other episodes are transferred from the *Amores* in so mechanical and lifeless a manner. For a detailed comparison see Elizabeth Thomas, 'Ovid at the Races', in *Hommages à Marcel Renard*, ed. J. Bibauw, vol. I (*Collections Latomus* 101 (1969)), pp. 710–24.

**135. nobilium . . . certamen equorum :** cf. *Am.* iii. 2. 1 'non ego nobilium sedeo studiosus equorum.' The breeding of racehorses had already been reduced to a fine art, and an expert might reel off whole pedigrees without a slip ('memoriter totam equini generis sobolem computantem', [Cyprian], *de Spectaculis* 5). But to the Christian writer all was vanity: 'quam uana sunt ipsa certamina, lites in coloribus, contentiones in curribus, fauores in honoribus, gaudere quod equus uelocior fuerit, maerere quod pigrior, annos pecoris computare, consules nosse, aetates discere, prosapiam designare, auos ipsos atauosque memorare' (ibid.).

**136. commoda :** providing a kind of link with 131–2. Compare also *Am.* iii. 2. 20, quoted on 157–8.

**137–8.** Such methods of communication are familiar in the elegists, particularly at drinking-parties (e.g. 569 ff.).

**139. proximus a domina nullo prohibente sedeto :** cf. *Tristia* ii. 284. Ovid mentions this as unusual. In the Circus Maximus men and women could sit together; in the theatre seating arrangements were segregated (109 n.). For the amphitheatre see 167 n.

**sedeto :** This archaic form of imperative suits the measured tone of a didactic work.

**141–2.** A line marks the space for each individual on the bench, but obviously the accommodation is cramped, so that everyone is wedged against his neighbour whether he likes it or not. Compare *Am.* iii. 2. 19–20 (quoted on 157–8).

**141. et bene, quod :** 'And what a good thing it is that . . .', cf. Quintilian, *Decl.* 307 'bene, quod magna scelera his ipsis, quibus occultari uidentur, aperiuntur', alternatively 'o bene' (ii. 605, Martial vii. 15. 3 'o bene, quod silua colitur Tirynthius illa!').

**si nolis :** 'whether one likes it or not'. The second person must be generalizing, as the lover should not lack enthusiasm.

**143. hic :** 'at this juncture'. Do not rush into intimacies straight away, but start with some everyday remarks (*publica uerba*,

144) about the racing. After 147 your actions become more pointed.

**145–6.** Since we have not yet had the ritual procession which opens the games (147–8), these lines may refer to a preliminary parade of contestants.

**145. studiose :** 'as if you were a fan'—you are not genuinely interested in racing (cf. *Am.* iii. 2. 1) but merely support the same team as the girl (146). Compare Petronius 52 'in argento plane studiosus sum; habeo scyphos urnales . . .', Plautus, *Miles Gloriosus* 802 (a man without hobbies) 'qui nisi adulterio studiosus rei nulli aliaest'.

Of course 'studiose' is vocative, not adverb; similar is Tibullus i. 7. 53 'sic uenias hodierne' (see Smith ad loc. and Nisbet and Hubbard on Horace, *Odes* i. 2. 37). With such an accomplished technician as Ovid I would be reluctant to plead metrical exigency alone. He may be imitating Hellenistic experiments such as Callimachus fr. 599 ἀντὶ γὰρ ἐκλήθης Ἴμβρασε Παρθενίου.

**147–8.** Before the actual races, statues of the gods are carried round the Circus in procession (cf. Tertullian, *de Spectaculis* 7), and the people show their devotion by applauding individual gods. From *Amores* iii. 2. 45 ff. it would appear that each man gave especial applause to his patron deity—sailors to Neptune, soldiers to Mars etc. Naturally the lover claps Venus (148, cf. *Am.* iii. 2. 55–6). When Caesar took the unprecedented step of adding his own statue to the procession (cf. Suetonius, *Divus Julius* 76) Cicero expressed his delight that the people withheld the customary applause even from Victory, who was carried next: 'populum uero praeclarum, quod propter malum uicinum ne Victoriae quidem ploditur!' (*ad Att.* xiii. 44. 1).

**147. caelestibus . . . eburnis :** ivory statues of the gods. Daremberg and Saglio s.v. Circus, fig. 1528, give a representation of the *pompa* in which the statues of Cybele and Victory can be seen, carried on the shoulders of bearers. Ivory may be thought surprisingly grand for this occasion, but Kenney compares Tacitus, *Annals* ii. 83. 2, Suetonius, *Titus* 2, Dio xliii. 45. 2.

Without doubt 'caelestibus . . . eburnis' is the right reading, although some older editors accepted the remarkable variant 'certantibus . . . ephebis', referring it to the Troy Game (cf. *Aeneid* v. 545–603). See Kenney, *CR* N.S. 3 (1953), 7–10; he discusses the manuscript tradition fully, and establishes the superiority of 'caelestibus . . . eburnis' on the ground of sense. For we want some reference to the statues of the gods to introduce 148; also *ephebus* is used by Latin writers of the classical period only (a) of Greek (or sometimes foreign) youths, most often as an exact equivalent for the technical term ἔφηβος, or (b) pejoratively, with a suggestion of effeminacy.

**149–62.** *There are all kinds of small services which you may perform for the girl. You can pick any specks of dirt off her clothing* (149–52), *lift up her dress if it trails on the ground* (153–4), *rebuke the man behind for sticking his knees into her back* (157–8). *Even smoothing a cushion, fanning her or slipping a stool under her feet can win gratitude* (159–62).

Almost all these precepts have been extracted from *Amores* iii. 2. 21–42, but with an unmistakable loss of charm (see on 157–8).

**149–50.** Compare *Am.* iii. 2. 41–2 'dum loquor alba leui sparsa est tibi puluere uestis: / sordide de niueo corpore puluis abi!' Removing specks from another's clothing was traditionally a mark of the Flatterer (Aristophanes fr. 657, Theophrastus, *Characters* 2).

**149. utque fit :** 'as will happen'.

**153–4.** Compare *Am.* iii. 2. 25–6 'sed nimium demissa iacent tibi pallia terra: / collige, uel digitis en ego tollo meis.'

**153. pallia :** The *pallium* was a Greek cloak, worn by, amongst others, *hetaerae* both Greek and Roman; cf. Cicero, *de Div.* ii. 143 'amica corpus eius texit suo pallio.'

**157–8.** It is worth dwelling a little longer on the parallel from *Amores* iii. 2. 19–24 (for 19–20 cf. 136 and 141–2 above):

> quid frustra refugis? cogit nos linea iungi;
>   haec in lege loci commoda Circus habet.
> tu tamen, a dextra quicumque es, parce puellae:
>   contactu lateris laeditur illa tui;
> tu quoque, qui spectas post nos, tua contrahe crura,
>   si pudor est, rigido nec preme terga genu.

The *Amores* passage has considerably more bite; in 21–2 Ovid rebukes the man on the other side for sitting too close to the girl—just what he is doing himself, and in any case nobody can help it (19–20). Also there is pleasing irony in the indignant 'si pudor est' (24), and the scornful 'quicumque es' (21) loses its force in the *Ars* (157).

**159. fuit utile multis :** 'many people have found it beneficial', a keynote of the *A.A.*, which is supposed to be based on tested and proved methods (29). The same idea is often expressed by 'profuit' (e.g. 161), which we also find in Virgil's *Georgics*, as in i. 84 'saepe etiam steriles incendere profuit agros', iv. 267 (cf. Kenney in *Ovidiana*, p. 203). This touch is most at home in didactic poems on medicine (e.g. Nicander, *Theriaca* 926, 935 and *ad nauseam* in the *Liber Medicinalis* of Serenus Sammonicus).

**160. puluinum :** a cushion.

**161.** Compare *Am.* iii. 2. 37–8 'uis tamen interea faciles arcessere uentos, / quos faciet nostra mota tabella manu?'

  **tabella :** normally taken to be a fan. But the word does not seem to recur in this sense, so perhaps it is an ordinary writing-tablet used as an improvised fan.

**162. scamna** : a foot-stool.

**163–70.** *Finding a girl at a gladiatorial display.*

Ovid makes no comment on the shows themselves beyond 'sollicito' (164 n.); here his characteristic flippancy is less than pleasing. The problem had worried Cicero ('crudele gladiatorum spectaculum et inhumanum non nullis uideri solet, et haud scio an ita sit, ut nunc fit' *Tusc. Disp.* ii. 41), but his attitude remains ambivalent; he particularly disliked the modern refinements of contests with animals (*ad Fam.* vii. 1. 3), but saw in the traditional man-to-man encounter a prime example of how training can overcome the fear of death (*Tusc. Disp.* ii. 41). Seneca is the first surviving Roman writer to condemn the carnage unequivocally (e.g. *Epist.* 95. 33). Early Christian authors were also firm in their opposition (Tertullian, *de Spectaculis* 19, cf. Augustine quoted on 166).

**164. sparsaque sollicito tristis harena foro** : cf. Propertius iv. 8. 76 'nec cum lasciuum sternet harena forum', *Tristia* ii. 282. Under the Republic gladiatorial displays took place in the Forum Boarium, and later in the Forum Romanum. Statilius Taurus built the first stone amphitheatre in 29 B.C., but even after then shows were occasionally given in the Forum.

**sparsa . . . harena** : Sand would be strewn over the central area, to make it level and to absorb blood.

**sollicito** : not a general epithet of a forum, but applying only to this occasion. It could refer as much to the anxiety of spectators that their favourite should win as to the suffering of the gladiators.

**165. illa saepe puer Veneris pugnauit harena** : Michael Grant (*Gladiators*, p. 96) mentions artistic portrayals of Cupids fighting as gladiators. This unsavoury idea looks like a Roman twist to the Greek figure of Love as a wrestler (Gow on Theocritus 1. 97–8—see further on 232). Whether it could have any basis in the grotesque mock-fights (*prolusiones*, see Seneca, *Epist.* 7. 3) which provided comic relief between serious encounters in the arena I do not know (cf. iii. 515). Gladiators also might take names like Ἔρως or Cupido (Versnel, *Mnemosyne* 1974, 369 n. 13).

**166. et, qui spectauit uulnera, uulnus habet** : Ovid may be adapting a line of argument used against gladiatorial displays (cf. 99 n.)—that they brutalized the spectators no less than the competitors (e.g. Seneca, *Epist.* 7. 3–5, contrast Cicero, *Tusc. Disp.* ii. 41). Augustine tells us about his friend Alypius who was taken to a show against his will be some fellow students, and left, at least temporarily, an addict: 'percussus est grauiore uulnere in anima quam ille in corpore, quem cernere concupiuit, ceciditque miserabilius quam ille, quo cadente factus est clamor' (*Conf.* vi. 8).

**uulnus habet :** When a gladiator was wounded, the people would cry out 'habet' or 'hoc habet', 'he has got it!'( e.g. Terence, *Andr.* 83). Compare Servius on *Aeneid* xii. 296.

**167. dum loquitur tangitque manum poscitque libellum :** Is the young man attracting the girl's attention to ask if he can borrow her programme? In that case he must be sitting next to her. But Suetonius (*Div. Aug.* 44) clearly states that the emperor only allowed women to watch gladiatorial displays from the back seats (cf. 109 n., 139 n. for the theatre and the Circus). Maybe rules were not so tight when the show was in the Forum (164). Alternatively this line may not concern the girl: perhaps our hero is chatting casually, greeting a friend (tangitque manum) or buying a programme, and only catches sight of his Waterloo at 169 'saucius ingemuit.'

**libellum :** cf. Cicero, *Phil.* ii. 97 'tanquam gladiatorum libellos palam uendident'; these would be sheets giving the name of each fighter. On the publicity for such shows, see Michael Grant, *Gladiators*, pp. 63–4.

**168. posito pignore :** Betting was quite regular, as on the chariot-races (e.g. Martial xi. 1. 15, Juvenal 11. 201).

**169. telum...uolatile :** Cupid's arrow. The phrase is traditional epic, first surviving in Sueius fr. 8 Morel (see Pease on *Aeneid* iv. 71).

**170. muneris :** the technical term for a gladiatorial display.

**171–6.** *How many young men fell in love at the mock sea-battle which the emperor recently put on!*

This was a re-creation of the Battle of Salamis (172) fought on an artificial lake on the right bank of the Tiber. A specially con-structed aqueduct, the *Aqua Alsietina* (see Nash, *Pictorial Dictionary*, vol. I figs. 27–8), brought water for the lake, and thirty large vessels together with numerous smaller ones were engaged, involving three thousand gladiators, not counting the oarsmen (*Res Gestae* 23). The site was used later by Nero and Titus for sea-battles (Martial, *Liber Spectaculorum* 28. 1–2 'Augusti labor hic fuerat committere classes / et freta nauali sollicitare tuba'), but Martial (ibid. 11–12) is confident that Titus' show of A.D. 80 will eclipse all previous ones:

> Fucinus et diri taceantur stagna Neronis:
> hanc unam norint saecula naumachiam.

Traces of the Naumachia were still visible in the time of Alex-ander Severus (Dio lv. 10); see further Platner and Ashby s.v. *Naumachia Augusti.*

**171. modo :** The sea-battle formed part of the festivities at the dedication of the temple of Mars Ultor, vowed by Octavian at Philippi 'pro ultione paterna' (Suetonius, *Div. Aug.* 29). This temple was dedicated on 1 August, 2 B.C. (Dio lx. 5 is clear on the date), and the sea-battle must have occurred about the same time—celebrations went on for several days. Some modern authorities give 12 May, 2 B.C. for the dedication of Mars Ultor, but this seems to rest on a confusion with other games honouring Mars (cf. *Fasti* v. 551 ff.). I am grateful to Mr. E. W. Gray for information here.

From this and the following section on Gaius' eastern campaign, we may conclude that books i–ii of the *Ars* were published late in 2 B.C. or early in 1 B.C. There is no very cogent reason for thinking that Ovid inserted the passages in a second edition (see further Introduction p. xiii).

**172. Persidas induxit Cecropiasque rates :** These naval spectaculars would represent combats between famous fleets of the past; thus Julius Caesar showed 'Tyrians' against 'Egyptians' (Suetonius, *Div. Julius* 39) and Claudius 'Sicilians' against 'Rhodians' (*Div. Claud.* 21). Here we have a re-creation of the Battle of Salamis, more ambitious since the right side had to win (Dio lv. 10 'the Athenians were victorious on that occasion as well').

**Cecropias :** 'Athenian', from the mythical king Cecrops.

**173. ab utroque mari :** 'from the Eastern and Western shores of the world', cf. *Met.* xv. 829–30 'gentisque ab utroque iacentes / Oceano', Virgil, *Georgics* iii. 33, Propertius iii. 9. 53. Compare Martial on Titus' games in A.D. 80 (*Liber Spectaculorum* 3. 1–2) 'Quae tam seposita est, quae gens tam barbara, Caesar, / ex qua spectator non sit in urbe tua?'

Some interpret 'from the Adriatic and Tuscan seas' (often called the 'mare superum' and 'mare inferum'). But the sentiment 'from all over Italy' is too tame, and does not match up to 'ingens orbis' (174).

**174. ingens orbis in Urbe fuit :** Juxtaposing 'urbs' and 'orbis' was a favourite trick, particularly in encomia of Rome; see Otto, *Sprichwörter*, s.v. *Urbs*, Joseph Vogt, *Orbis Romanus*, p. 17 n. 3, E. Bréguet in *Hommages à Marcel Renard*, ed. J. Bibauw, vol. I (*Collections Latomus* 101 (1969)), pp. 140–52. Surely the most elegant expression was in Rutilius Namatianus, *de Reditu Suo* i. 66 (to the goddess Roma) 'urbem fecisti quod prius orbis erat.' Today it survives in the Papal 'Urbi et Orbi'. As to the vast crowd, Suetonius writes of an earlier display 'tantum undique confluxit hominum ut plerique aduenae aut inter uicos aut inter uias tabernaculis positis manerent, ac saepe prae turba elisi exanimatique sint plurimi et in his duo senatores' (*Div. Jul.* 39).

**176. aduena . . . amor :** reminiscent of Euripides, *Hippolytus* 32 ἐρῶσ’ ἔρωτ’ ἔκδημον.

**177–228.** *Finding a girl at a military triumph.*

Ovid's chief inspiration lies in Propertius iii. 4 (lines 11–18 quoted on 217 ff.). But only at 219 does he start to advise the young man how to behave when watching a triumphal procession together with his girlfriend; the previous lines contain a *propempticon*, or send-off poem, for young Gaius Caesar, soon to leave for the East. Just a few common features of a *propempticon* are observed, e.g. a prayer to the gods for the traveller's safety and success (203–4), a promised offering upon his return (205), and the joyful anticipation of festivities when the wanderer rejoins his countrymen (213 ff.). Statius, in writing a much more formal *propempticon* for Maecius Celer (*Silvae* iii. 2), used Ovid as one of his models (on the type, see Francis Cairns, *Generic Composition in Greek and Roman Poetry* (Edinburgh 1972), particularly chs. 1 and 9, and Nisbet and Hubbard on Horace, *Odes* i. 3). Interestingly, we have another *propempticon* written for Gaius at the same time by Antipater of Thessalonica (translated and discussed in my Appendix III); the latter seems to have lived in Rome, and his work shows several points of contact with Ovid, so one poet may be consciously imitating the other.

The ultimate cause of Gaius' expedition lay in troubles over Armenia. Not long before the pro-Roman king Artavasdes had been expelled, together with Roman troops supporting him, by Tigranes III. Things were made worse by the accession of a new king in Parthia, Phraates V, usually known as Phraataces, who gave assistance to Tigranes and did not seem disposed to compromise. Official Roman sources speak either of a revolt by Armenia ('desciscentem et rebellantem' (*Res Gestae* 27)) or of aggression by Parthia (Velleius ii. 100 'Parthus desciscens a societate Romana adiecit Armeniae manum').

Since Ovid has his eye on the disputed Parthian succession (195–200), Phraataces deserves a fuller notice. He was the son of Phraates IV by an Italian slave-girl Musa (or Thermusa) whom Augustus had presented to the king. This lady determined to secure the throne for her son, and, according to Josephus, was instrumental in persuading Phraates to send his four legitimate sons to Rome (probably not in 20 B.C. when the standards of Carrhae were surrendered, but some time later, about 10 B.C.). So Phraataces was being groomed for power, but, as Josephus remarks drily (*A.J.* xviii. 42), he found it boring to await the course of nature, and, following established family custom, had his father murdered. Tetradrachms of Phraataces are known with dates approximating to July, August, and September, 2 B.C.,

# EXPLANATION OF PLATE I

(a) Aureus of Augustus, struck at Lugdunum between 5 February 2 B.C. (when Augustus became officially Pater Patriae—see note on line 197) and 31 December 1 B.C. (after which Gaius entered his consulship).

Obverse: CAESAR AVGVSTVS DIVI F PATER PATRI-
AE
Head of Augustus, laureate, to right.

Reverse: C L CAESARES AVGVSTI F COS DESIG
PRINC IVVENT
Gaius and Lucius standing, facing.

The Reverse inscription and the brothers' equipment may be illustrated by Augustus' words in *Res Gestae* 14 'equites autem Romani uniuersi principem iuuentutis utrumque eorum parmis et hastis argenteis donatum appellauerunt' (compare Ovid line 194). My colleague Mr. J. G. Griffith kindly allowed me to reproduce this fine specimen from his collection.

(b) Silver Tetradrachm of Phraataces (Phraates V), struck at Seleucia on the Tigris. As usual with kings of Parthia, he bears the dynastic name 'Arsaces'. Dated Hyperberetaios 310 of the Seleucid era, approximately September 2 B.C. For Phraataces see further on lines 177 ff. and 195–200.

Obverse: Bust of Phraataces to left, with pointed beard. He wears diadem, earring, beaded necklace, and cuirass.

Reverse: ΒΑCΙΛΕΩC ΒΑCΙΛΕΩΝ ΑΡCΑΚΟΥ ΕΥΕΡΓΕΤΟΥ ΔΙΚΑΙΟΥ ΕΠΙΦΑΝΟΥC ΦΙΛΕΛΛΗΝΟC ('Of Arsaces, King of Kings, the Benefactor, the Just, the god-made-manifest, the Phil-hellene').

Phraataces enthroned to right, receiving diadem from Tyche of city. In field ΙΤ (310); in exergue [Υ]ΠΕΡΒΕΡΕΤΑ[ΙΟC]
This coin is in the British Museum.

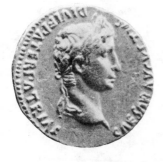
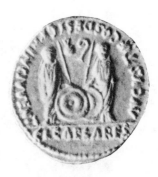
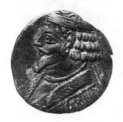
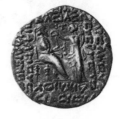

I. Contemporary coins relevant to *Ars Amatoria* I

  (a) Aureus of Augustus (twice natural size)
  (b) Silver tetradrachm of Phraataces (natural size)

*For detailed explanation, see page 66*

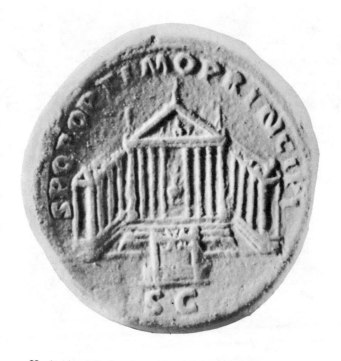

II. A coin of Trajan showing the temple of Venus Genetrix
(reconsecrated by him), with the portico of the Forum
Iulium and in front the Appiades fountain. Ovid describes
exactly this scene in lines 79 ff.

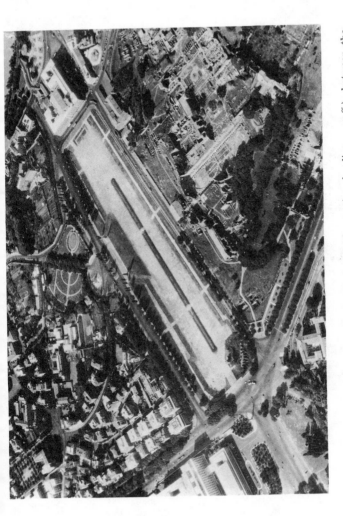

III. Aerial photograph of the Circus Maximus (the setting for lines 135 ff.), between the Aventine and the Palatine

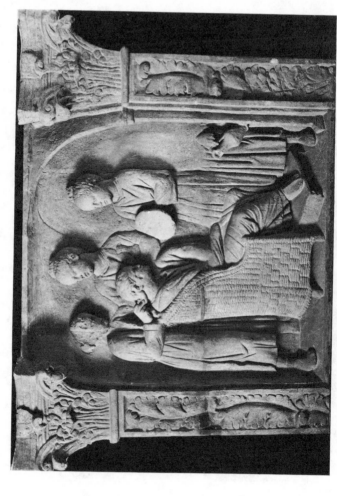

IV. 'Matutinos pectens ancilla capillos' (367). Relief from a tombstone. III Century A.D.

while an isolated British Museum coin (which Mr. D. G. Sellwood kindly re-examined) appears to be of April 2 B.C. Strangely enough Velleius Paterculus, an eyewitness of the eventual meetings between Gaius and Phraataces, thought the young Parthian king impressive (ii. 101 'iuuene excelsissimo').

Neither affairs in Armenia nor the usurpation of Phraataces were tolerable to Augustus—he must have hoped that one of the four hostage-princes whom he had entertained so lavishly in Rome (Strabo xvi. 1. 28) would make a compliant king of Parthia. But dealing with the situation was another matter. He himself had grown too old and feeble to take the field, and Tiberius was sulking in Rhodes. So with great reluctance he appointed his grandson (and adopted son) Gaius, child of Marcus Agrippa and Julia, and elder brother of Lucius and Agrippa Postumus. While preparations for the campaign went ahead, there were diplomatic exchanges between the two principals. Phraataces through an embassy explained the position as he saw it and asked for the return of his half-brothers the hostages—not, I imagine, inspired by any brotherly love, but to remove possible rivals whom Rome might set up against him. Augustus replied by letter with a command for the Parthian to withdraw from Armenia and to abandon the title of king, which suggests that Rome had indeed planned to install one of the four hostage-princes on the Parthian throne (a point confirmed by Ovid in lines 195 and 198, if my interpretation is correct). Phraataces, however, was not abashed and wrote back styling himself 'King of Kings'. So preparations for war continued (all this from Dio lv. 10).

Ovid more than once writes as if the object of the campaign were to conquer the whole Parthian empire (177–8, 202). Such language had been quite regular in the poetry of fifteen to twenty-five years before (e.g. Horace, *Odes* iii. 5. 4, Propertius iii. 1. 16, iii. 4, iv. 6. 79–84), but may surprise us at this date when the lost standards of Carrhae were safely back in Rome, restored through negotiation, and the Roman and Parthian realms had apparently settled down to a comfortable coexistence. There was talk of extending the campaign to Arabia (Pliny, *N.H.* vi. 141, 160). Juba, the scholarly king of Mauretania, fired Gaius' imagination by writing on the natural history of the area (Pliny, *N.H.* xii. 56 'Iuba rex in iis uoluminibus quae scripsit ad C. Caesarem Augusti filium ardentem fama Arabiae'), and Dionysius (?Isidore) of Charax treated the geography (ibid. vi. 141). Even Augustus fostered the young man's ambition, wishing him 'the popularity of Pompey, the daring of Alexander and his own good fortune' (Plutarch, *Moralia* 207e).

Did all this reflect public enthusiasm or the genuine intentions of the emperor? Such a question is very hard to answer. The idea of a grand Eastern campaign to rival the exploits of Alexander and avenge Carrhae once and for all must have had considerable appeal; clearly the return of the standards did not altogether assuage the feeling that Rome had a score to settle with Parthia. On the other hand Crassus had left for the East amid tribunician curses (Dio xxxix. 39) and the re-introduction of conscription was always feared (Velleius ii. 130). P. A. Brunt in a noteworthy review article (*JRS* 53 (1963), 170–6) argues that we should not dismiss too lightly the poets' words about Eastern conquest, and that they may genuinely have reflected the intentions of Augustus even though he was never free to undertake such an expedition. But what most strikes me about this occasion, when a Roman force actually did campaign in the East, is the ludicrous disparity between the language heralding the event and the final outcome. Not that Gaius tried and failed to defeat the Parthians—he never came to grips with them at all (*Remedia Amoris* 155–6 must obviously be taken with a pinch of salt). In A.D. 1, the year of his consulship, he may have fought in the region of Arabia (see James Zetzel, *GRBS* 11 (1970), 259–66, T. D. Barnes, *JRS* 64 (1974), 22–3, and J. I. Miller, *The Spice Trade of the Roman Empire* (Oxford, 1969), pp. 15–16, for the theory that he destroyed the port of Aden). Next spring the trouble with Parthia was resolved amicably enough at two working dinner-parties, first on Roman and then on Parthian territory (Velleius ii. 101). Both sides made concessions: Phraataces was recognized as king, but his half-brothers stayed in Rome, whence one of them, Vonones, came to rule Parthia briefly about A.D. 8–12. Even Tigranes of Armenia, after making humble supplication to Rome, was granted the throne which he already held. No sign of any Roman disappointment with this outcome can be detected; Augustus duly describes Armenia as 'domitam per Gaium filium meum' (*Res Gestae* 27). Therefore the whole affair, in my opinion, is most plausibly viewed as a great propaganda exercise for an expedition that was never meant to do much more than show the flag. To finish the story: after meeting Phraataces Gaius became involved in another Armenian disturbance, and received a wound from which he eventually died (21 Feb., A.D. 4). Thus he never returned victorious to fulfil Ovid's prophecy. Nor did Phraataces reign for long; if identical with the 'Phraates son of Phraates' in *Res Gestae* 32, he may have ended his career as a suppliant of Augustus.

Our poet's tone is fulsome (but hardly rivalling Antipater's (Appendix III)), interspersed with characteristic touches of sharpness and humour (e.g. 211, 227–8). In the panegyric parts

I suspect the influence of Hellenistic court-poetry addressed to
the king as a god, a type of composition which has perished
almost entirely, but we may get some idea of it from epigrams
dedicated to the Roman imperial house by Greek poets like
Antipater of Thessalonica, Crinagoras, and Philip (all in Gow–
Page, *The Garland of Philip*). The question of the emperor's
divinity was a tricky one in Rome and Italy; Ovid here avoids
the worst excesses which other poets and later he himself
sometimes indulged in. He also shows some tact over the future
position of Gaius (194). Finally there is just the right division
between the parts assigned to Augustus and to Gaius in the
coming campaign (see on 177). Nobody could pretend that this
is one of the most notable pieces in Ovid, but I myself find it less
embarrassing than many similar utterances in Augustan verse.
Recently it has become fashionable to portray Ovid as a definite
anti-Augustan—a picture hard to reconcile with these lines.
We need not take his enthusiasm at face value, but Galinsky
(*WS* 1969, 97 ff.) may err in the other direction.

**177. Caesar :** Augustus, as the prime mover of the expedition,
rather than Gaius, the actual commander. The emperor himself
was unable to take the field because of frailty and advancing age
(Dio lv. 10. 18); at 191–2 (see note) Ovid pictures him command-
ing through Gaius. On the other hand 'dux meus' (202) clearly
does refer to Gaius.

 **domito quod defuit orbi :** 'the part remaining before we are
masters of the world'. The language is not untypical; cf. Horace,
*Epist.* i. 18. 57 (Augustus) 'siquid abest Italis adiudicat armis'.
Understand 'nobis' with 'addere' (178, cf. 202). Line 671
'quantum defuerat pleno post oscula uoto?' rather favours
keeping these words as a self-contained unit, although Kenney
would now consider punctuating 'domito, quod defuit, orbi /
addere', making the expression more like Horace, *Odes* ii. 9. 21–2
'Medumque flumen, gentibus additum / uictis'.

**179–82.** Propertius in 16 B.C. gave a specimen of what the patri-
otic poet should be composing (iv. 6. 79–84), from which Ovid has
taken several hints:

> hic referat sero confessum foedere Parthum:
>  'reddat signa Remi, mox dabit ipse sua:
> siue aliquid pharetris Augustus parcet Eois,
>  differat in pueros ista tropaea suos.
> gaude, Crasse, nigras si quid sapis inter harenas;
>  ire per Euphraten ad tua busta licet.'

Line 82 contains a remarkable anticipation: Gaius and Lucius
had been adopted as mere infants in 17 B.C.

**179. Crassi gaudete sepulti :** The triumvir M. Licinius Crassus and his son Publius (hence the plural) met their death in the desert near the Mesopotamian town of Carrhae (53 B.C.). Ovid is presumably making the same point as Propertius (above), that the region where they perished will now become part of the Roman empire. Poetic licence neglects the fact that Crassus never received burial (Val. Max. i. 6. 11).

**180. signa :** In 20 B.C. the Parthians had restored the legionary eagles lost at Carrhae, together with others taken from subordinates of Antony (cf. *Res Gestae* 29, Velleius ii. 91); passages like this show how much and how long the memory rankled. The standards had particular cause for joy at the time of writing (2 B.C.), since they had just been transferred to the new temple of Mars Ultor (171 n., cf. *Res Gestae* 29), henceforth to be the starting-point of generals going on foreign campaigns (Dio lv. 10. 2)—a fact which 'ultor adest' (181) might recall to Ovid's first readers. Compare *Fasti* v. 595, where the temple of Mars Ultor is connected with the avenging both of Julius Caesar and of Crassus.

**181. ducem profitetur :** 'claims the title of commander', not unlike 127 'comitemque negarat'.

**183 ff.** I feel that Hellenistic court-poetry must lie somewhere in the background (see introduction to this passage). Ovid shows more moderation than the Greek poets (e.g. 'child of Zeus' in Antipater (Appendix III), cf. Gow–Page on Crinagoras, *Anth. Pal.* ix. 562. 6 = Crinagoras no. 24, G–P, *The Garland of Philip*). Emperor-worship in Ovid is discussed by Kenneth Scott in *TAPA* 61 (1930), 43–69, but he does not allow for any progression in the language used; only after the exile does our poet throw off all restraint when speaking of the emperor's divinity.

**183.** There must have been Romans who were worried by Gaius' lack of experience; indeed Augustus appointed him with great reluctance (Dio lv. 10. 18).

**184. Caesaribus uirtus contigit ante diem :** no doubt thinking of Octavian himself, who had commanded in the civil war before he was twenty (cf. Tacitus, *Annals* xiii. 6).

**185–6.** For the doctrine compare Callimachus, *hymn* 1. 55–7 καλὰ μὲν ἠέξευ καλὰ δ' ἔτραφες, οὐράνιε Ζεῦ, / ὀξὺ δ' ἀνήβησας, ταχινοὶ δέ τοι ἦλθον ἴουλοι. / ἀλλ' ἔτι παιδνὸς ἐὼν ἐφράσσαο πάντα τέλεια ('Fair was your growth, and fair your nurturing, heavenly Zeus. Quickly did you come to manhood and swiftly your beard grew. But even as a child you planned everything to perfection'). This may have been a conventional method of praising a young ruler; Callimachus himself probably has one eye on Ptolemy Philadelphus, who, like Zeus, supplanted elder brothers. Later we find precocious maturity among the themes of imperial panegyric in prose (e.g. *XII Panegyrici Latini* (Mynors) 4. 7 'inuolucra infantiae uiuidum rupit ingenium ').

**185. ingenium caeleste :** avoiding too crude a presentation of Augustus and/or Gaius as a god. Like 'diuinus', 'caelestis' can express enthusiasm without implying actual divinity, e.g. Cicero, *Phil.* v. 28 'illas caelestis diuinasque legiones '.

**187–90.** Hercules and Bacchus are quoted for their precocity. But other parallels with the young Gaius also strike one: (a) both were demi-gods who through their benefits to men achieved full divinity (Cicero, *de Legibus* ii. 19, Horace, *Odes* iii. 3. 9 ff.), (b) they were far-ranging conquerors (compared to Augustus in *Aeneid* vi. 801 ff.), (c) Bacchus had campaigned in the East (190). Victorious Roman generals, like Hellenistic kings before them, might take on the symbols of Bacchus or Hercules, e.g. Marius (Pliny, *N.H.* xxxiii. 150, cf. *N.H.* vii. 95 on Pompey). Much material can be found in Dorothea Michel, *Alexander als Vorbild für Pompeius, Caesar und Marcus Antonius* (Collections Latomus 104, 1967).

**187–8.** Juno, always jealous of her husband's offspring by mortal women, had sent two monstrous snakes in the night against the infant Hercules, but he strangled both with his bare hands.

**188. pressit :** 'strangled' (literally 'squeezed').

**et in cunis iam Ioue dignus erat :** Any comparison of Hercules to Gaius and Jupiter to Augustus is extremely oblique. Yet contemporary Greeks regularly spoke of the emperor as Zeus (see on 183 ff.), and the same applies to Ovid in exile (see K. Scott, *TAPA* 61 (1930), 52–8).

**189–90.** Euripides (*Bacchae* 15) had described Dionysus leaving 'the walled towns of Bactria'. The myth of his Indian conquest gained impetus in the Hellenistic period, gradually being assimilated to the exploits of Alexander (see A. D. Nock, *JHS* 48 (1928), 21–30). It is the subject of the longest surviving Greek epic, the *Dionysiaca* of Nonnus (*c.* 5th cent. A.D.) in 48 books; no doubt epics had been written earlier on the same theme (e.g. the *Bassarica* of Dionysius, from which we have fragments).

**189. nunc quoque qui puer es :** an ingenious bit of sophistry—like Apollo, Bacchus is ever young (e.g. *Met.* iv. 18 'tu puer aeternus'). Called by T. B. L. Webster (*Hellenistic Poetry and Art*, p. 1) 'peculiarly the god of the Hellenistic age', he appears in contemporary art as a delicate youth (e.g. Webster, op. cit., p. 23).

**190. cum timuit thyrsos :** The ivy-wreathed wand (*thyrsus*), wielded by an ecstatic Maenad with the aid of the god's supernatural power, became a more deadly weapon than sword or spear (see Dodds on Euripides, *Bacchae* 113).

**191–2.** The connection of thought appears to be: *after all we need not worry about Gaius' youthfulness because he will have the moral* *authority* (cf. 'auspiciis') *and maturity* (cf. 'annis') *of Augustus behind him.* It is true that the compliment to Gaius is lessened, but throughout Ovid keeps a careful balance between praising Gaius and praising Augustus (cf. Galinsky, *WS* 1969, 98–9).

Here the emperor seems almost to be commanding through Gaius. Such a manner of speaking finds several parallels in the latter part of his principate, e.g. Horace, *Odes* iv. 14. 33–4 'te copias, te consilium et tuos / praebente diuos'. Particularly striking is *Tristia* ii. 173–6, where Tiberius, the actual commander in the field, is presented as little more than a puppet: 'per quem bella geris, cuius nunc corpore pugnas, / auspicium cui das grande deosque tuos, / dimidioque tui es praesens et respicis urbem, / dimidio procul es saeuaque bella geris'. Statements like this were meant to increase the (none too high) military reputation of the *princeps* by proxy.

**191. auspiciis . . . patris:** Originally a Roman commander took the omens in person before battle; the technical phrase for a holder of *imperium* himself leading an army was 'ductu auspiciisque' (Pliny, *N.H.* iii. 136, cf. Ogilvie on Livy iii. 1. 4). But when, as here, the general was only the legate of a magistrate with *imperium*, the auspices would be those of his superior; compare e.g. Tacitus, *Annals* ii. 41 'ductu Germanici, auspiciis Tiberii'. Also implicit is the idea that a campaign 'under the auspices of Augustus' must inevitably be successful because of the moral authority of the *auspex* (cf. *Tristia* ii. 174 quoted above).

**annisque:** i.e. the experience and wisdom represented by Augustus' years. So Paul Turner translates the line: 'This boy general will have his father's age and authority behind him.' *Tristia* ii. 229 pays the reverse compliment to Augustus, 'nunc te prole tua [Tiberius] iuuenem Germania sentit.' Such a combination of youthful vigour and seasoned judgement is often stressed in panegyric, e.g. Pliny, *Pan.* 8. 4 (Nerva and Trajan), *XII Pan. Lat.* 7. 13. 5 (Maximian and Constantine).

Alan Ker (in *Ovidiana*, p. 224), supported by Kenney, took Ovid to mean that Gaius will be victorious at the same tender age at which Octavian won his first successes. But then the coupling of 'annis' with 'auspiciis' (which Ker misrepresents) surely becomes impossibly awkward—the *present* auspices but the *past* age of his father. True, the youthfulness of Octavian in his first command was a *topos*; the place, however, where we are meant to recall it is line 184.

**192.** The typical repetition throws emphasis on 'uinces', which is picked up by 'tale rudimentum' in 193.

**193.** 'Such is the first campaign (i.e. a victorious one) which we expect from you under the tutelage of so great a name.'

**rudimentum** : as often, a technical term for one's first military service.

**tanto sub nomine** : The 'great name' is Augustus himself; cf. *Tristia* ii. 442 'quis dubitet nomina tanta sequi?' and Owen ad loc. Alternatively he might mean 'because you bear so great a name' (that of Caesar), but the use of *sub* is not so easy to parallel (see, however, Housman's *Manilius* i, p. lxxi).

194. **nunc iuuenum princeps** : In 5 B.C. Gaius had been saluted by the Equites as 'Princeps Iuuentutis', a title also conferred on his younger brother Lucius in 2 B.C. (cf. *Res Gestae* 14, Tacitus, *Annals* i. 3 and the Augustan coin in my Plate III).

**deinde future senum** : Undoubtedly Augustus hoped that one of the brothers would succeed to his position in full; witness the private letter preserved by Gellius, *N.A.* xv. 7. But Ovid's antithesis 'iuuenum—senum' suggests for Gaius the impeccably Republican title of 'Princeps Senatus' ('senator' being connected with 'senex') which Augustus held for over forty years (*Res Gestae* 7). One can see here tact, ingenious evasiveness, or even a regard for constitutional propriety. Contrast two less guarded statements: (a) on a centurion's altar set up to the brothers (*I.L.S.* 137) 'nam quom te, Caesar, tempus exposcet deum . . . / . . . sint hei tua qui sorte terrae huic imperent', (b) posthumous honours for Gaius at Pisa (*I.L.S.* 140 = Ehrenberg–Jones, *Documents Illustrating the Reigns of Augustus and Tiberius*², no. 69) 'iam designatum . . . principem' (in spite of appearances, not an official phrase).

195-6. 'Since you yourself have brothers [Lucius and Agrippa Postumus], avenge brothers who have been wronged [the four Parthian hostage-princes supplanted by their half-brother Phraataces]; since you yourself have a father [Augustus], maintain a father's rights [the right of Phraates IV to choose which of his sons should succeed him].' On the historical background, see my introduction to this passage. I am grateful to Mr. E. W. Gray, also to Dr. L. A. Holford-Strevens and others at the Oxford Philological Society for help here. The argument is sophistical but typically sharp: Gaius, who exemplifies family loyalty ,concord, and dutifulness, should punish Phraataces for his flagrant lack of these qualities. This interpretation gives real force to the *cum*-clauses (perhaps its decisive merit).

Almost all commentators and translators assume that 'fratres ulciscere laesos' and 'iura tuere patris' denote Gaius' brothers and Gaius' father. But, while he could reasonably be urged to maintain the rights of Augustus, it would be bizarre in the extreme to describe events in Parthia and/or Armenia as a personal injury to Lucius and Agrippa Postumus. Finally, *Prosopographia Imperii Romani*, s.v. Erato (probably depending

78 COMMENTARY

on *Res Gestae*, ed. Mommsen², p. 114), refers 'fratres ulciscere laesos' to Tigranes III of Armenia and his sister-wife Erato— does this at least imply a correct understanding of 'cum tibi sint fratres'? But Erato apparently did not abdicate till A.D. 1 after the death of Tigranes, while Ovid writes in late 2 B.C. or early 1 B.C., and in any case Tigranes III, as we have seen, was originally opposed by Rome.

**197–200.** A contrast in filial devotion, picking up 196 'iura tuere patris'.

**197. genitor patriaeque tuusque :** Augustus had long been known as 'pater patriae' unofficially (Horace, *Odes* i. 2. 50). But the title was not formally conferred on him until 5 February 2 B.C. —the year in which this passage was written. So there would be special point in the compliment here. Suetonius (*Div. Aug.* 58) quotes the actual words of Messala Corvinus in proposing the honour: 'quod bonum faustumque sit tibi domuique tuae, Caesar Auguste! sic enim nos perpetuam felicitatem rei publicae et laeta huic precari existimamus: senatus te consentiens cum populo Romano consalutat patriae patrem.' For linking the two types of parenthood cf. Pliny, *Pan.* 10. 6 (on Nerva and Trajan) 'ita ille nullo magis nomine publicus parens, quam quia tuus'.

**198.** 'Your enemy [Phraataces] took the throne by force from his father [Phraates IV].' See on 177 ff. and 195–6.

inuito : implying not merely that Phraates IV was unready to hand over power, but furthermore that he never wished Phraataces to succeed him, preferring another of his sons. While this insinuation seems doubtful (to judge from Josephus, *A.J.* xviii. 42), it would suit the Roman aim of replacing Phraataces with one of the hostage-princes.

**199. tu pia tela feres, sceleratas ille sagittas :** each side designated by its most typical weapon, as at Statius, *Silvae* iii. 2. 126 'Eoas iaculo damnare sagittas'. A Roman would probably refer 'tela' to the heavy legionary javelin (*pilum*) which symbolized Roman power; cf. Lucan, *Bellum Ciuile* i. 6–7 'pila minantia pilis' and x. 47–8. In reality Gaius would no more carry a *pilum* than would the Parthian king fight as a light-armed horse-archer (see on 209–10).

**200. iusque piumque :** 'Justice and Devotion', cf. *Heroides* 8. 4.

**202. Eoas Latio dux meus addat opes :** The whole of the East was proverbially wealthy—above all Arabia, thought to be among the targets of Gaius. For commercial profit as an acknowledged aim of Eastern conquest, cf. Propertius iii. 4. 1–3 'arma deus Caesar dites meditatur ad Indos . . . / magna, uiri, merces', and, more lightheartedly, Horace to Iccius (*Odes* i. 29).

**203. Marsque pater :** as the father of Romulus (though Greek inscriptions call Gaius both 'son of Ares' and 'the new Ares',

*I.G.* III. 1. 444 and 444a). Mars also had a special connection with
the *gens Iulia* (see Nisbet and Hubbard on Horace, *Odes* i. 2.
36), and, *qua* Mars Ultor, with this campaign (see on 180).

   **date numen eunti :** 'grant him your power as he goes'. Ovid
rather jumps the gun in attributing 'numen' to Augustus
(Cicero happily spoke of the Senate's 'numen', i.e. the authority
and dignity, but 204 shows that the word must bear a fuller
sense here). After the exile he does this without qualms, e.g.
*Tristia* v. 3. 45–6 'flectere tempta / Caesareum numen numine,
Bacche, tuo.' Towards the end of Augustus' reign Tiberius
dedicated an Ara Numinis Augusti (? A.D. 5 or A.D. 9, cf. L. R.
Taylor, *AJP* 58 (1937), 185–93, D. Fishwick, *Harvard Theo-
logical Review* 62 (1969), 356–67). For emperor-worship in Ovid
generally, see Kenneth Scott, *TAPA* 61 (1930), 43–69.

**204.** The line could well be printed in brackets, for it explains (and
in Augustus' case half apologizes for) 'numen' in 203.

   **alter eris :** Such was the orthodox doctrine. After his death
Augustus would enter the company of heroic individuals like
Hercules who won deification by their services to mankind
(Horace, *Odes* iii. 3. 9–16).

**205 ff.** Ovid proposes to write an epic poem as his personal offer-
ing for the victory and safe return of Gaius (205). This will be
a *Bellum Parthicum*, describing the glorious campaign. To write
epics on individual wars was a Roman tradition stretching back
to the *Bellum Poenicum* of Naevius; Augustan examples in-
cluded the *Bellum Actiacum* by Rabirius and the *Bellum Siculum*
by Cornelius Severus, on the wars of Octavian against Antony
and Sextus Pompey respectively (see further Owen on *Tristia* ii.
529). Gaius, of course, never returned to Rome, but in any case one
cannot for a moment take Ovid's proposal seriously. Light poets
were always just about to pen a martial epic when some god
providentially dissuaded them (for the *recusatio* see Nisbet and
Hubbard on Horace, *Odes* i. 6). Even to cry 'I will, I will' and
then not to do it can be taken as a sophisticated version of the
*recusatio*; by merely outlining the themes which he would like to
handle, the poet avoids having to treat them at length (e.g.
Propertius ii. 10, iii. 9. 47 ff.). Furthermore Parthian campaigns
were recognized as a forbidding subject: 'neque enim quiuis
horrentia pilis / agmina nec fracta pereuntis cuspide Gallos /
aut labentis equo describat uulnera Parthi' (Horace, *Sat.* ii. 1.
13–15, cf. Persius 5. 4).

   For this section our poet may have taken some hints from the
complex proem to Virgil's third *Georgic* (1–48). There Virgil
looks forward to an epic in which Octavian would be the central
figure ('in medio mihi Caesar erit', 16); it was to contain battles
('ardentis . . . pugnas', 46) and a victory over Parthia ('addam

urbis Asiae domitas, pulsumque Niphaten, / fidentemque fuga
Parthum uersisque sagittis', 30–1). See L. P. Wilkinson, *The
Georgics of Virgil*, pp. 165–72 and his Appendix III. There is one
great difference between Virgil and Ovid: Virgil, because of his
ties with the regime, may have been under some pressure to cele-
brate military victories, but the same cannot be true of Ovid.
These lines represent nothing but a *jeu d'esprit*.

**205. uotiuaque carmina reddam :** In the normal manner of a *pro-
pempticon* he vows an offering for the wanderer's safe return—
his poem. Compare Statius, *Silvae* iii. 2. 131–2 'quanta uotiua
mouebo / plectra lyra.' Statius' *propempticon* for Maecius Celer
echoes Ovid several times (cf. particularly 213 n.).

**206. et magno nobis ore sonandus eris :** denoting a grandiloquent,
epic style. Compare Horace, *Sat.* i. 4. 43–4 'os / magna sona-
turum', Virgil, *Georgics* iii. 294 'magno nunc ore sonandum',
and for the 'magnum os' also Propertius ii. 10. 12. The ex-
pression may go back beyond Horace and Virgil (? to Ennius).
In Greek similar is Callimachus fr. 757 φθέγγεο κυδίστη πλειοτέρῃ
φάρυγι (see Pfeiffer's note).

**207. aciemque meis hortabere uerbis :** perhaps a hit at the un-
reality of many speeches attributed to a general before battle.
For some of the conventional topics in a *paraceleusis*, see Ogil-
vie on Livy iii. 61.

**208.** 'May the words which I give you be worthy of your spirit!'

**209–10.** The Parthian manœuvre of shooting from a feigned
retreat, which looms so large in Roman literature, was in fact
traditionally Asian (cf. Plutarch, *Crassus* 24. 6). Malcolm
Colledge (*The Parthians* (Thames & Hudson 1967), pp. 38–9)
reproduces graffiti of the Parthian light-armed horse archer,
and also of the mailed lance-bearing cavalryman who resembled
a medieval knight.

**209. tergaque Parthorum Romanaque pectora :** suggesting (though
not very seriously) that the Roman is brave and simple, his foe
cowardly and devious. Romans honoured a 'uulnus aduersum',
received in face of the enemy (e.g. Cicero, *de Or.* ii. 124, *in
Verrem* v. 3), but a wound on the back showed that you must
have been running away. The annoying point about the Par-
thian tactic was that it combined safety with honour, as Plu-
tarch reflects (*Crassus* 24. 6).

**211.** 'Since flight is your way to victory, what will remain for you,
Parthian, in defeat?' One might have thought the Parthian
shaft exhausted as a fruitful literary theme. Ovid perhaps
deserves credit for a new twist (also 216), but one shudders to
imagine a martial epic (see on 205 ff.) written along these lines.
For the form of expression compare proverbs like 'when water
chokes you, what can you wash it down with?' (Aristotle, *E.N.*

vii. 1146a35), 'if the salt have lost his savour, wherewith shall it be salted?' (Matthew 5: 13).

**213–28.** *The triumph of Gaius.* For details of a Roman triumph, with illustrations, see Daremberg and Saglio, s.v. *Triumphus*; the younger Pliny pictures a triumph of Trajan as part of his *Panegyric* (17).

**213. ergo erit illa dies, qua tu :** cf. Statius, *Silvae* iii. 2. 127–8 'ergo erit illa dies qua te maiora daturus / Caesar ab emerito iubeat discedere bello.' One finds many such phrases in prophecy, e.g. ἔσσεται ἦμαρ ὅτ' ἄν (*Iliad* vi. 448), ἥξει καιρὸς ἐκεῖνος (Theocritus 23. 33, cf. Headlam on Herodas 4. 50), 'scilicet et tempus ueniet' (*Georgics* i. 493). The tone is normally solemn, and often doom-laden; here rather it is jubilant. Anticipation of festivities at the traveller's return formed a regular part of the *propempticon* (cf. *Amores* ii. 11. 45 ff., Statius, *Silvae* iii. 2. 133 ff.).

**pulcherrime rerum :** a surprisingly informal mode of address, cf. Horace, *Sat.* i. 9. 4 'quid agis, dulcissime rerum?' The genitive 'rerum' means literally 'in the world'.

**214. quattuor in niueis . . . equis :** The triumphator would ride in a quadriga drawn by four snow-white horses; cf. Tibullus i. 7. 8, Propertius iv. 1. 32, Daremberg and Saglio, s.v. *Triumphus* figs. 7095 and 7097.

**aureus :** He wears the triumphal *toga picta*, crimson liberally spangled with gold embroidery (see Mayor on Juvenal 10. 38); also the chariot is gilt. For the favourite Ovidian contrast of colours (aureus—niueis) see my note on *Met.* viii. 9.

**215. ibunt ante duces :** with a typical edge. One expects leaders to go in front of their men, but here they do so in chains. Commanders of the defeated people might be kept alive for the triumph and preceded the triumphator either on foot or in a chariot (Daremberg and Saglio, fig. 7094). Normally they were led away to be executed when the procession reached the foot of the Cliuus Capitolinus.

**217 ff.** This picture of the lover with his girlfriend watching a triumph may be inspired by Propertius iii. 4, particularly lines 11–18:

> Mars pater, et sacrae fatalia lumina Vestae,
> ante meos obitus sit precor illa dies,
> qua uideam spoliis oneratos Caesaris axis,
> ad uulgi plausus saepe resistere equos,
> inque sinu carae nixus spectare puellae
> incipiam et titulis oppida capta legam,
> tela fugacis equi et bracati militis arcus,
> et subter captos arma sedere duces!

Compare also Horace, *Odes* iv. 2. 41 ff.

**218. diffundetque animos :** 'will release the spirits'. This use of the verb is paralleled by διαχέω in Greek.

**219.** Only here does Ovid start to advise the young man how to behave at a triumph, thus justifying the section which began at 177.

**220. quae loca, qui montes, quaeve ferantur aquae :** cf. Tacitus, *Ann.* ii. 41 'uecta spolia captiui simulacra montium fluminum proeliorum'. There might be lists, personifications (as with rivers) or even pictures showing conquered territory. Josephus provides one of our fullest descriptions of a Roman triumph, that of Vespasian and Titus (*B.J.* vii. 132 ff.). He mentions tableaux three or four storeys high, representing episodes in the war; part of his account can be paralleled from the Arch of Titus (see Ernest Nash, *Pictorial Dictionary of Ancient Rome*, s.v. Arcus Titi).

    **ferantur :** carried by bearers on a litter (*ferculum*).

**221–2.** Answer all her questions, and be prepared to volunteer information as well, reeling off the names with an air of complete confidence even if you are making them up.

**223–4.** Colossal statues of river-gods, usually reclining on one elbow, were familiar in Roman art. We can distinguish a personification of the river Jordan on the Arch of Titus, and Father Danube on Trajan's Column.

**223. praecinctus harundine frontem :** just as the actual river is fringed with reeds. Compare *Met.* ix. 3 of Achelous 'inornatos redimitus harundine crines'.

**224. coma . . . caerula :** cf. Homer's epithet for Poseidon, κυανο-χαίτης ('dark-locked').

    **dependet :** in mourning.

    **Tigris erit :** 'that must be the Tigris'. For the future cf. *Amores* i. 2. 7 'sic erit: haeserunt tenues in corde sagittae.'

**225. hos facito Armenios :** a general mass of undistinguished prisoners.

    **haec est Danaeia Persis :** The Persian kings were supposed to derive from Perses, son of Perseus and Andromeda; Perseus was a son of Danae by Zeus. The myth appears in Herodotus (vii. 150) and might well have interested Hellenistic writers.

    **Persis :** properly the Achaemenid province of Parsa, stretching south and west from Persepolis. At this time Persis was ruled by kings nominally dependent on Parthia who preserved many Achaemenid traditions, and from Persis came the Sasanian dynasty which was to overthrow the Parthians early in the third century.

**228. si poteris, uere, si minus, apta tamen :** a pleasant ending, reminiscent of Seneca's 'uetulus nomenclator qui nomina non reddit sed imponit' (*Epist.* 27. 5). If you do not know their names, invent something suitably complex and colourful.

**229–52.** *Finding a girl at a party*. A banquet is one of the favourite
settings for love-elegy, but here Ovid will not advise the young
man how to behave (as at 565 ff.). These are still early days—
only at 265 does the poet assume that you have found the ideal
girl—and he is more concerned to point out the dangers of
making a hasty choice. For the wine and the artificial lighting
both tend to rob one of that clear judgement which is the essence
of *ars* (246, 249–50).

**230. est aliquid :** for the reticence cf. *Amores* iii. 2. 83, Propertius
ii. 33. 42.

**231–6.** Difficult lines which have caused great trouble to com-
mentators. E. J. Kenney (*CQ* N.s. 9 (1959), 244–6) provides an
extremely valuable elucidation of the motifs from both Greek
and Roman poetry, and goes a long way towards dispelling the
obscurity (my notes are much indebted to him). See also the
discussion of Kenney by F. W. Lenz in the Commentary to his
Berlin 1969 edition (which does not add anything very sub-
stantial), and by H. Tränkle in *Hermes* 100 (1972), 393–6.
Finally, Elaine Fantham, *Comparative Studies in Republican
Latin Imagery* (1972), 82–91, has a useful collection of material,
chiefly from Comedy.

Part of the obscurity is due to constant playing on two levels,
a favourite Ovidian turn (see my note on *Met.* viii. 549 ff.).
Bacchus may be a horned god at one moment, and at the next
simply wine, by metonymy—or even both at once (see on 231
'positi'). Cupid appears first as a winged boy, then as love in the
heart of a young man (236). Further difficulties centre around
lines 234 and 235, which on the most reasonable interpretation
of the allegory might seem contradictory (see ad locc.). There I
would guess that Ovid was preoccupied with the visual image of
the winged god caught in a slightly glutinous liquid and striving
to free himself, but at the same time he could not resist adding
various conventional ideas about love, the symbolism of which
was not wholly consistent. Kenney speaks of Ovid's deficient
visual imagery, and suggests that he may have failed to visualize
clearly what he was describing. This could be right in the pre-
sent case, though I would contend that Ovid's visual imagina-
tion was generally first-class.

We need not, however, convict the poet of incompetence.
There is quite a sophisticated way of writing in which the visual
imagery may be fragmented, confusing, or even provocatively
absurd. As an example of the last, consider the neoteric conceit
mocked by Persius (1. 94) 'qui caeruleum dirimebat Nerea
delphin', where readers are surely meant to conjure up momen-
tarily a picture of a dolphin parting the sea-god himself, be-
fore rejecting it as ridiculous. I suspect that the technique is

primarily neoteric. Propertius' images often shift alarmingly
and produce no coherent picture (see Gordon Williams on iv. 11,
*Tradition and Originality in Roman Poetry*, p. 393); it may be
significant that similar difficulties have been felt in Propertius
ii. 12, an allegorical account of the attributes of Cupid.

Kenney well quotes from the *Anacreontea* (5 Bergk) an erotic
allegory concerning Love and wine which in atmosphere has
a striking affinity to Ovid:

> στέφος πλέκων ποθ᾽ εὗρον
> ἐν τοῖς ῥόδοις Ἔρωτα.
> καὶ τῶν πτερῶν κατασχὼν
> ἐβάπτισ᾽ εἰς τὸν οἶνον·
> λαβὼν δ᾽ ἔπινον αὐτόν,
> καὶ νῦν ἔσω μελῶν μου
> πτεροῖσι γαργαλίζει.

('Once when I was plaiting a garland, I found Love among the
roses. Holding him fast by the wings, I dipped him in wine and
took and drank him down. Now inside my body he is tickling me
with his wings.')

**231-2.** Kenney suggests plausibly enough that this couplet may
derive from a painting which showed Cupid and Bacchus
wrestling, while 233-6 look like Ovid's own rhetorical exploita-
tion. A struggle between Cupid and Bacchus is familiar in the
context of drowning one's sorrows, but then Bacchus will win
(e.g. Lygdamus (*Corpus Tibullianum* iii. 6. 4) 'saepe tuo cecidit
munere uictus Amor').

**231. positi :** in a double sense (see above). The god reclines on a
couch and the wine is set down on a table. We need not consider
Lachmann's 'poti'.

    **teneris . . . lacertis :** something of an oxymoron—*lacertus*
usually implies brawn and muscle.

    **adducta :** cf. *Met.* ix. 52 (another wrestling match) 'adducta-
que bracchia soluit'.

**232. purpureus . . . Amor :** The epithet indicates a brilliant sheen
(cf. Horace, *Odes* iv. 1. 10 'purpureis . . . oloribus') and is often
applied to a youthful complexion, e.g. *Aeneid* i. 590-1 'lumen-
que iuuentae / purpureum'.

    **Bacchi cornua pressit :** Cupid 'forces down' (more than 'holds
fast' (Kenney)) the horns of Bacchus, as in wrestling with a
bull. Compare *Met.* x. 83-4 'depressaque dura / cornua figit
humo' (with Gardiner, *JHS* 26 (1906), 16-17, figs. 7-8), Calli-
machus fr. 258 θηρὸς ἐρωήσας ὀλοὸν κέρας. For Love as a wrestler see
Kenney's parallels and Pearson on Sophocles fr. 941. 13 τίν᾽ οὐ
παλαίουσ᾽ ἐς τρὶς ἐκβάλλει θεῶν; The bull-form belongs to Bacchus not

as god of wine, but in a more primitive conception of him as god
of untamed power (see Dodds's *Bacchae*, pp. xi–xx).

**233–4.** Love has overcome Wine in wrestling, but in the process
his wings are drenched so that for the moment he cannot fly
away. Profiting from the accident, Love takes possession of a
young man's heart.

**233. bibulas :** 'absorbent'.

**234. permanet et capto stat grauis ille loco :** a paradox. Love is
held fast by the drenching of his wings, but makes a virtue out
of necessity and captures the territory where he is trapped
(a young man's heart). For the literary motif, see on 235.

> **grauis :** Kenney discerns as many as three meanings present
here—(1) 'with wet garments', (2) *uino grauatus*, (3) 'trouble-
some', cf. Theocritus 3. 15 βαρὺς θεός.

**235. pennas . . . excutit :** I think Kenney must be right in saying
that here Love flies away (he does not merely 'shake out' his
wings to dry them). 'Excutit' is equivalent to the simple
'quatit' (cf. 22). The poet appears to mean that passion inspired
by wine is impermanent and lasts just so long as the intoxi-
cation which gave it birth (Kenney). But would this not contra-
dict line 234 (*permanet* and *capto . . . loco*)?

I have suggested that Ovid may have been intrigued by the
picture of the winged god hastening to free himself from the
wine. Also he seems to play with two opposing literary motifs.
One stressed the difficulty of shaking off a painful love, e.g.
Propertius ii. 12. 15 'euolat heu nostro quoniam de pectore
nusquam', Meleager 10 Gow–Page (*Anth. Pal.* v. 212). 5–6
ἐφίπτασθαι μέν, Ἔρωτες, / οἶδατ', ἀποπτῆναι δ' οὐδ' ὅσον ἰσχύετε;, while the
other symbolized the fickleness of love, e.g. ii. 19–20 'et leuis est
et habet geminas, quibus auolet, alas; / difficile est illis imposu-
isse modum' or Moschus' poem entitled 'Love the Runaway'
(1 Gow). Debaters might argue on either side whether or not
Cupid was rightly credited with wings (see Butler and Barber
on Propertius ii. 12).

**236.** 'Cupid, as he flies away, shakes the wine off his wings; the
wine is still tinged with love, so that the god leaves some traces
of himself behind, and the lover does not get off heart-whole
(*nocet*) . . . Even the transitory passion inspired by wine cannot
evaporate without leaving some mark behind' (Kenney). Kenney
also gives parallels for love conceived as a liquid (even a poison)
dripped into the heart, although our passage is not quite
typical.

> **et :** Just a few drops can be dangerous.

**237–44.** *Wine prepares the heart for love; it removes all worries and
inhibitions, making men behave in a completely natural way.* From
the innumerable parallels (cf. Nisbet and Hubbard on Horace,

*Odes* i. 18) one may quote Horace, *Odes* iii. 21. 13–20, a passage
which Ovid had particularly in mind (239 n.):

> tu lene tormentum ingenio admoues
> plerumque duro; tu sapientium
>   curas et arcanum iocoso
>     consilium retegis Lyaeo;

> tu spem reducis mentibus anxiis
> uiresque et addis cornua pauperi
>   post te neque iratos trementi
>     regum apices neque militum arma.

**237.** For the proverbially close connection (Otto, *Sprichwörter*, s.v.
*Venus*) between love and wine cf. Callimachus, *Ep*. 42 Pf. 3
ἄκρητος καὶ Ἔρως μ᾿ ἠνάγκασαν, Propertius i. 3. 13–14 'et quamuis
duplici correptum ardore iuberent / hac Amor hac Liber, durus
uterque deus.'

**238. diluiturque mero** : oxymoron.

**239. tum pauper cornua sumit** : echoing Horace, *Odes* iii. 21. 18
(quoted above). Horns symbolize courage and pugnacity (cf.
Otto, s.v. *Cornu* 4)—the poor man will not allow himself to be
pushed around. We find the same figure in Greek (Diogenianus
vii. 89 κέρατα ἔχειν· ἐπὶ τῶν ἀνδρείας ὑπόληψιν ἐχόντων).

**241–2.** According to L. P. Wilkinson (*Ovid Recalled*, p. 133) the
couplet sounds 'innocently Tibullian', and one may agree. But
he surely errs in adding 'The *simplicitas* (alias *rusticitas*) is
modesty, and the *artes* are the girl's defences.' These are not
moral terms; Ovid merely says that wine strips away every-
thing that hides a person's underlying character.

  **aeuo rarissima nostro / simplicitas** : because contemporary
Rome was polished and sophisticated, the hall-mark of the times
being *cultus* (iii. 127). Simplicitas sounds like a goddess who
only occasionally manifests herself—indeed Ovid may be think-
ing of Aratus on Justice in the Silver Age (*Phaenomena* 115 ff.,
a celebrated passage).

**242. deo** : of course Bacchus.

**243. animos iuuenum rapuere puellae** : The hunters have become
the hunted, highlighting the dangers of finding a girl at a party.

**244. ignis in igne** : cf. Otto, *Sprichwörter*, s.v. Ignis 3, Diogenianus
vi. 71 μὴ πῦρ ἐπὶ πῦρ.

**245–52.** *Before becoming too closely involved with a girl, be sure to
examine her in the daylight, as you would before buying a jewel or
a dyed woollen garment.*

  The antithesis between lamp-light and sunlight was to some
extent proverbial (Otto, s.v. Sol 5). I wonder whether Ovid is not
giving a new turn to conventional abuse of those who hid them-

selves away in banquets—this would be very much in his man-
ner (cf. 99 n., 166 n.). As Cicero puts it (*pro Caelio* 67) 'lux
denique longe alia est solis, alia lychnorum.' The poet agrees,
but for an unexpected reason.

**245. nimium ne crede lucernae** : an echo (perhaps unconscious) of
Virgil, *Ecl.* 2. 17 'nimium ne crede colori.'

**246. iudicio formae** : pointing forward to the Judgement of Paris
in 247–8, lines typical of Ovid's ability to extract a novel point
from even the most hackneyed myth.

**247 ff.** Notice how *luce* (247), *nocte* (249) and *diem* (252) are all
emphatically placed at the beginning or end of a line.

**249–50.** Naturally he mentions the wine and artificial light as an
advantage when advising the opposite sex: 'etsi turpis eris,
formosa uidebere potis, / et latebras uitiis nox dabit ipsa tuis'
(iii. 753–4).

**251.** Also perhaps proverbial was the sentiment that bargains
should be made in broad daylight; cf. Euripides, *Cyclops* 137
ἐκφέρετε· φῶς γὰρ ἐμπολήμασιν πρέπει.

    **de tincta murice lana** : The ability to distinguish between dyed
materials of different quality became a standard example of
good judgement; cf. Horace, *Epist.* i. 10. 26–7 'qui Sidonio
contendere callidus ostro / nescit Aquinatem potantia uellera
fucum', Quintilian xii. 10. 75 'ut lana tincta fuco citra purpuras
placet' citing Ovid fr. 5 Morel, cf. *Remedia* 707–8.

**253–62.** *But places where females congregate are more numerous
than grains of sand on the sea-shore.* The poet ends this section
with two examples of the many places which he could have
added—Baiae (255–8) and the grove of Diana at Aricia (259–62).

**254. numero cedet harena meo** : see Nisbet and Hubbard on
Horace, *Odes* i. 28. 1 'numeroque carentis harenae'. 'Cedet
harena' may contain a secondary playful idea of the sand
yielding under a heavy weight, as in 'inposito cessit harena
pede' (560).

**255. Baias** : the fashionable spa on the north shore of the Bay of
Naples, surrounded by villas of the rich. Baiae was endowed
with superb scenery and a pleasant climate; cf. Horace, *Epist.* i.
1. 83 'nullus in orbe sinus Bais praelucet amoenis', Martial xi.
80. But it acquired a persistent reputation for immorality.
Varro wrote a satire entitled *Baiae*; there, according to him,
'non solum innubae fiunt communes, sed etiam ueteres puella-
scunt' (*Saturarum Menippearum* p. 105 Riese). Cicero feared that
sober-minded jurymen might be prejudiced against a youth 'qui
Baias uiderit' (*pro Caelio* 27), and Propertius (i. 11) was worried
by the dangers to which Cynthia exposed herself there. But
nobody wrote more pungently than Martial, on the lady who
'Penelope uenit, abit Helene' (i. 62. 6).

**praetextaque litora Bais :** As Kenney says, the repetition
'Baias . . . Bais' throws emphasis on 'litora', the notorious
beaches; the reading 'Bais' has the support of Y as well as O.
All the same, I prefer (like older editors) the variant 'uelis', 'the
shore fringed with sailing-boats'; cf. *Aeneid* vi. 4–5 'litora
curuae / praetexunt puppes' and Lucan x. 537. These small
pleasure boats were a prominent feature of Baiae (Juvenal 12.
80 'Baianae . . . cumbae', Seneca, *Epist.* 51. 12 'tot genera
cumbarum uariis coloribus picta', Propertius i. 11. 9–10, cf.
Horace, *Odes* iv. 15. 3–4). Ovid's practice in a quick review such
as we have here is to pack the maximum amount of vivid
detail into the minimum of space (cf. 256, 259–60); on this score
'uelis' is superior to 'Bais'.

A grammatical point (noted by Kenney) might also be taken
to favour 'uelis'. After 'praetextaque litora', of course 'uelis'
would be ablative, but 'Bais' must be dative, and the dative is
not apparently associated with 'praetexo' until Silver Latin
(though Kenney quotes Cicero, *de Re Publica* ii. 9 for a dative
with 'adtexo').

**256. et quae de calido sulphure fumat aqua ? :** Compare Propertius
iii. 18. 2 'fumida Baiarum stagna tepentis aquae'. The hot
sulphur-springs had earned the town its previous name of
Aquae Cumanae (Livy xli. 16).

**257. uulnus . . . in pectore :** Some waters were thought particu-
larly good for wounds (cf. Pliny, *N.H.* xxxi. 6, xxxi. 17). Here,
however, the man who came for a cure leaves with a different
sort of trauma.

**259–62.** The grove of Diana Nemorensis at Aricia lay about ten
miles south of Rome along the Appian Way (cf. *suburbanae*,
259). This cult was extremely rich and popular, involving a
torch-light procession of women which Propertius' Cynthia had
often attended (ii. 32. 9–10).

**260. partaque per gladios regna nocente manu :** The extraordinary
conditions of priesthood at Aricia provided the starting-point
for Sir James Frazer's great anthropological work *The Golden
Bough* (vol. I, ch. 1—see also his index s.v. Aricia and note on
*Fasti* iii. 271). The priest was called 'king of the grove', 'Rex
Nemorensis' (cf. *regna*); on priestly kings, see *The Golden
Bough* vol. I, ch. 2. He had to be a runaway slave, and won the
office by slaying his predecessor in single combat.

Clearly the custom looked back to a primitive age and manner
of thought. Frazer (on *Fasti* iii. 271) summarized his thesis
argued at length in *The Golden Bough* thus: 'Kings are possessed
of a divine or magical character in virtue of which not only the
welfare of their subjects but the course of nature . . . are bound
up with the life of the ruler and will suffer serious damage, or

even perish, if his strength fails through illness or old age. . . .
To avert these dangers various measures are adopted. Some-
times the king's reign is limited to a period during which he may
reasonably be expected to retain his bodily and mental vigour.
. . . Sometimes, without putting a fixed term to his reign and his
life, his people allow him to reign till symptoms of old age or
serious illness warn them of his threatened dissolution. . . .
Sometimes, again, he is suffered to reign and to live so long as
he can give proof of undiminished health and strength by repel-
ling any armed attacks made upon him by candidates for the
throne.'

Did such a barbarous rite really take place in Ovid's day? The
answer seems to be in the affirmative. Strabo's chilling picture of
the priest gazing around with drawn sword, ever fearful of an
attack (v. 3. 12), suggests an eye-witness. The priest in Cali-
gula's reign had survived for many years—possibly evidence
of relaxation?—a fact which displeased the mad emperor:
'Nemorensi regi, quod multos iam annos poteretur sacerdotio,
ualidiorem aduersarium subornauit' (Suetonius, *Gaius* 35).
Pausanias in the second century A.D. (ii. 27. 4) implies that the
custom had lasted until his lifetime.

**261. quod est uirgo :** according to Kenney 'although she is a
virgin'. That would be a legitimate use of 'quod', which is
basically a colourless word ('as for the fact that') deriving its
sense, causal, conditional, or concessive, from the context (see
M. E. Taylor, *Yale Classical Studies* 12 (1951)', 229–49). But I
take Ovid to mean that precisely *because* Diana is a virgin and
opposed to Cupid, she delights to inflict on the people a *painful*
love (cf. 262 'uulnera').

**263–8.** *Recapitulation, and introduction to the second part of the
subject—how to catch the girl once you have found her.*

**263–5. hactenus . . . nunc :** echoing the start of *Georgics* ii, '*hac-
tenus* aruorum cultus et sidera caeli: / *nunc* te, Bacche, canam'
(see on 35–40). The same pattern can be found in almost any
other didactic poet, e.g. Lucretius iii. 31 ff. 'et quoniam docui
. . . / hasce secundum res . . .', Manilius iii. 160 ff. 'et quoniam
. . . exegimus . . . / nunc . . . canendum est', [Oppian], *Cyn*. iii. 1 ff.
ἀλλ' ὅτε δὴ κεραῶν ἠείσαμεν ἔθνεα θηρῶν / νῦν ἄγε . . . φράζωμεν . . .

**263. ubi retia ponas :** For the significance of the hunting metaphor,
see on 45–8. The 'nets of Venus' occur first in Ibycus, *Lyrica
Graeca Selecta* 267. 4 (further examples given by Kenney,
*Mnemosyne* 1970, 386–8).

**264. imparibus uecta . . . rotis :** another variation on what may be
termed Ovid's favourite joke—cf. *Amores* i. 1. 3–4 (Cupid steals
a foot from two hexameters, leaving an elegiac couplet), iii. 1. 8

(Elegy has one foot longer than the other). See on 39–40 for the chariot-image.

**Thalea** : simply 'my Muse'.

**267. dociles aduertite mentes** : the didactic poet's appeal for close attention from his audience, as in Lucretius iv. 912 'tu mihi da tenuis auris animumque sagacem', Manilius ii. 788–9, iii. 43 'nunc age subtili rem summam percipe cura.'

**268. fauens** : speaking only words of good omen, i.e. not speaking at all (like the Greek εὐφημεῖν). Here again we seem to be at a religious ceremony (cf. 30, 31).

**uulgus** : an ill-organized rabble, not yet instructed in the Art of Love; cf. iii. 46 of the women 'traditur armatis uulgus inerme uiris', Grattius, *Cyn.* i. 98 'ignarum . . . uolgus' of primitive hunters.

**269–350.** *First of all you must believe that the girl of your choice can be caught.* We expect Ovid to give instructions straight away, but instead here is the first of three long preliminary sections. Once more, the 'retardation' probably imitates didactic style (cf. 50 n.).

**271–2.** A figure particularly common in lighter forms of poetry, the ἀδύνατον or impossibility—'sooner will something against the laws of Nature happen than . . .' (see further on 747–8 and Nisbet and Hubbard on Horace, *Odes* i. 29. 10). We often find long strings of ἀδύνατα together, as at Horace, *Epodes* 16. 25–34 (rocks floating to the surface, rivers changing their course and mountains their position, fantastic unions between animals and concord between hostile species, terrestrial and marine creatures exchanging their abode).

**272.** For a reversal of fear and pursuit cf. Theocritus i. 135 καὶ τὰς κύνας ὤλαφος ἕλκοι, Lucretius iii. 751–2, Virgil, *Ecl.* 8. 53, [Virgil], *Dirae* 5 'delphini fugient pisces, aquilae ante columbas', Valerius Flaccus iii. 706.

**Maenalius . . . canis** : an Arcadian hound, reckoned among the best breeds (e.g. [Oppian], *Cyn.* i. 372).

**276. uir male dissimulat, tectus illa cupit** : a common doctrine—compare Euripides, *Andromache* 220–1 χεῖρον' ἀρσένων νόσον / ταύτην νοσοῦμεν, ἀλλὰ προύστημεν καλῶς ('we suffer more from this weakness than do men, but we conceal it decently') with P. T. Stevens's note.

**277. conueniat** : equivalent to a conditional—'should we males agree never to take the initiative . . .'. In 278 the future 'aget' is preferable to the subjunctive 'agat' (Kenney in *CQ* 1959, 246–7).

**279 ff.** *The violence of female passion*, proved first from the animal world (recalling a famous passage in Virgil's *Georgics*) and then from human examples.

**279:** Cf. Statius, *Silvae* iv. 5. 18 'nec uacca dulci mugit adultero.'

**280. femina cornipedi semper adhinnit equo** : cf. *Georgics* iii. 266 ff.,
a passage starting 'scilicet ante omnis furor est insignis equa-
rum', which Ovid echoes again at ii. 487–8.

**cornipedi** : Such compounds belong to the old epic style (cf.
on 20 'magnanimi'). This one survives first at *Aeneid* vi. 591,
vii. 779: the Greek prototype is not altogether clear, possibly
Homer's μῶνυξ (many Homeric epithets for horses are com-
pounded with πούς).

**281–2.** Compare Propertius iii. 19. 1–2 'obicitur totiens a te mihi
nostra ('of us men') libido: / crede mihi, uobis ('you women')
imperat ista magis' (followed by a mythological catalogue
containing some of the same *exempla* (Pasiphae, Myrrha,
Medea, Clytemnestra) as in Ovid). The argument is *a fortiori*:
if women can conceive so misguided a passion, how much more
confident should you be, dear reader, that you can win the girl
of your choice!

**283–342.** Something must be said about both the form and the
content of this passage, which may seem unattractive. First the
form: one can detect a certain resemblance to the so-called
'Catalogue-poem' or 'Collective-poem', a type, deriving from
the catalogue poetry ascribed to Hesiod, which became very
popular in the Hellenistic age; among its practitioners were
Hermesianax, Phanocles, and Euphorion. Such works would
gather together a large number of stories, told allusively in
different degrees of detail and perhaps differing styles. Virgil's
sixth *Eclogue* gives an indication of how this apparently arid
form might come to life in the hands of a master (see Gordon
Williams's perceptive analysis, *Tradition and Originality in
Roman Poetry*, pp. 243 ff.). In fact *Eclogue* 6 seems to have been
in Ovid's mind here no less than Propertius iii. 19: observe that
the story of Pasiphae is the only one treated in detail, and is
unevenly flanked by the others (being the third of ten *exempla*
in Ovid).

As to the content, these tales are uniformly morbid, describing
unnatural or even monstrous passions (this suits the argument,
see on 281–2). Here again we can discern a Hellenistic tendency;
a glance at Parthenius'*Love Romances*, prose summaries of myths,
many drawn from poets like Hermesianax and Euphorion, will
show the colouring. Indeed the subject of Orpheus' song at *Met.*
x. 153–4 almost suggests a recognized literary category:

inconcessisque puellas
ignibus attonitas meruisse libidine poenam.

The first two stories here (Byblis and Myrrha) have very strong
neoteric affiliations, though the later ones are at least as much
at home in Euripidean tragedy (see on 327 ff.). One should add

that the vagaries of female passion had aroused astonishment
and horror in male poets before the Hellenistic age (Aeschylus,
*Choephoroe* 494 ff.).

**283–4.** Byblis, daughter of Miletus, fell in love with her brother
Caunus. Ovid handles the myth at length in *Met.* ix. 447–665. It
appears also in some lines of Nicaenetus (fr. 1 Powell (*Collecta-
nea Alexandrina*), see Huxley, *Greek, Roman and Byzantine
Studies* 11 (1970), 251–7) and undoubtedly had a more extensive
Hellenistic background (Brooks Otis, *Ovid as an Epic Poet*,
pp. 386–8).

**284.** Like Myrrha in the next example, Byblis repents of her
infatuation. In making her hang herself Ovid follows Parthe-
nius, who in *Narr. Amat.* 11 quotes some mannered lines of his
own, ending καί ῥα κατὰ στυφελοῖο σαρωνίδος αὐτίκα μίτρην /
ἁψαμένη δειρὴν ἐνεθήκατο· ταὶ δ' ἐπ' ἐκείνῃ / βεύδεα παρθενικαὶ Μιλησίδες ἐρρήξαντο
('She hung her girdle from a hard oak, and into it inserted her
neck: over her did the daughters of Miletus rend their gar-
ments', fr. 29. 4–6 Martini).

**285–8.** Myrrha loved her father Cinyras and by him conceived
Adonis; after many wanderings she was transformed into a
myrrh-tree. The myth had connections with both Cyprus and
Arabia; once more it occurs in the *Metamorphoses* (x. 298–502,
see Brooks Otis, op. cit., pp. 391–2 for the sources). Most cele-
brated among earlier treatments was the formidably obscure
epyllion *Zmyrna* (another form of the girl's name) by Catullus'
friend Cinna (cf. Catullus 95).

**285. sed non qua filia debet :** The contrast between a daughter's
natural affection for her father and Myrrha's monstrous passion
appears frequently in *Met.* x; it may well derive from Cinna.

**286. et nunc obducto cortice pressa latet :** Notice two refinements
—Myrrha seems not so much transformed as enclosed within
the tree (somewhat like Propertius iii. 19. 16 'arboris in frondis
condita Myrrha nouae') and 'latet' pictures her hiding away in
shame (cf. *Remedia Amoris* 100 'non tegeres uultus cortice,
Myrrha, tuos'), an idea continued by 'lacrimis' in 287.

**287. illius lacrimis :** For Myrrha's tears perhaps compare Cinna
fr. 6 Morel 'te matutinus flentem conspexit Eous / et (read *te* a
second time?) flentem paulo uidit post Hesperus idem.' Appro-
priately they become after her transformation drops from the
myrrh-tree, as at *Met.* x. 499–500 'quae quamquam amisit
ueteres cum corpore sensus, / flet tamen, et tepidae manant ex
arbore guttae.' 'Lacrima', like δάκρυ, can in fact be used of the
exudation from any tree or plant.

**288. unguimur :** Concerning Rome's import of spices from the
East, see J. I. Miller, *The Spice Trade of the Roman Empire*
(Oxford, 1969), especially pp. 199 ff.

tenet : 'maintains', 'preserves', a common motif in trans-
formation-poetry; the change gives even a wicked person a kind
of immortality. Thus *Met.* x. 501-2 'est honor et lacrimis, stil-
lataque robore murra / nomen erile tenet nulloque tacebitur
aeuo.'

**289-326.** As mentioned before, Ovid's chief model for the Pasi-
phae episode lay in *Eclogue* 6. 45 ff. Virgil there writes in a neo-
teric style, delicately blending sentiment with irony; our poet,
no doubt intentionally, turns these elements into broad farce
and even black humour (such as when Pasiphae sacrifices any
good-looking cow which the bull seems to admire, 319-22). He
may also have an eye on the *Cretans* of Euripides, which con-
tained a notorious speech by Pasiphae defending herself (see
Page, Loeb *Greek Literary Papyri* (Poetry), pp. 70-6). One can
imagine the story of Pasiphae appealing to other neoteric poets,
but no clear evidence of their interest seems to survive (see,
however, on 305-6).

**289. nemorosae . . . Idae :** cf. Homer's epithet for the Trojan Ida,
ὑλήεσσα. Here, of course, the Cretan mountain of that name is in
question.

**290. candidus, armenti gloria, taurus :** For the word-order see
125 n. Only the position in a pentameter makes this example
slightly unusual.

**291. signatus tenui media inter cornua nigro :** We often find one
detail singled out like this, e.g. *Iliad* xxiii. 454-5 (a horse)
ὃς τὸ μὲν ἄλλο τόσον φοῖνιξ ἦν, ἐν δὲ μετώπῳ / λευκὸν σῆμα τέτυκτο περίτροχον
ἠΰτε μήνη, Horace, *Odes* iv. 2. 59-60 (a calf) 'qua notam duxit,
niueus uideri, / cetera fuluus'. See further Bühler on Moschus,
*Europa* 84-5.

   **media inter cornua :** a poetic cliché (see Pease on *Aeneid* iv.
61) but commentators never explain the phrase. It must mean
'midway between the horns'; the *cornua* themselves are not
*media*. Could the Latin start from something Greek, e.g. μέσον or
ἀνὰ μέσσον + genitive = in between?

**292. una fuit labes :** From a sacrificial point of view any spot
would be a blemish, disqualifying the animal. Contrast *Met.* xv.
130 'uictima labe carens'.

**293.** Both Cnossos and Cydonia were notable cities of Crete.

**296. inuida formosas oderat illa boues :** The point that Pasiphae's
bull would really much prefer a cow also occurs in Virgil (*Ecl.*
6. 55 'aut aliquam in magno sequitur grege'), but Ovid himself
has worked in the idea of her jealousy; he heightens both the
humorous and grotesque sides, even calling the rival cows 'pae-
lices' (320, 321).

**297. nota cano :** Callimachus has been much abused for writing
ἀμάρτυρον οὐδὲν ἀείδω ('I sing of nothing unattested', fr. 612), but

we should remember that the words may have applied only to a specific story in hand, like Ovid's parenthesis here.

**centum quae sustinet urbes :** glancing at the Homeric epithet for Crete, ἑκατόμπολις.

**298. quamuis sit mendax :** An old line ascribed to the Cretan philosopher Epimenides ran Κρῆτες ἀεὶ ψεῦσται, κακὰ θηρία, γαστέρες ἀργαί. This became proverbial: Saint Paul quotes it whole (Titus I : 12 'One of themselves, even a prophet of their own, said "The Cretans are always liars, evil beasts, slow bellies"') and others allude to it, e.g. Callimachus, *hymn* I. 8, Aratus, *Phaenomena* 30 (a Cretan story, 'if indeed it is true'), *Amores* iii. 10. 19 'Cretes erunt testes; nec fingunt omnia Cretes' (see Otto, *Sprichwörter*, s.v. Creta). G. L. Huxley (*Greek Epic Poetry from Eumelos to Panyassis*, pp. 81–2) would attribute the hexameter to *an enemy of* Epimenides, though such a melancholy reflection on his fellow countrymen does not seem impossible from the lips of the sage. Ovid gives the proverb an unexpected twist: here is no false story which the Cretans have invented for their own advantage, but a true and discreditable one which they cannot deny!

**299–300.** Pasiphae cuts choice fodder for the bull, but, not being a country type, she can scarcely do this competently. We are reminded of Apollo's problems when serving Admetus (Tibullus ii. 3. 17–20):

> o quotiens illo uitulum gestante per agros
>   dicitur occurrens erubuisse soror!
> o quotiens ausae, caneret dum ualle sub alta,
>   rumpere mugitu carmina docta boues!

**301–2. nec ituram cura moratur / coniugis :** cf. Propertius i. 8. 1, when Cynthia threatens to leave for Illyria, 'nec te mea cura moratur?'

**303 ff.** Virgil too turns to address the queen (*Ecl.* 6. 47 ff. 'a uirgo infelix, quae te dementia cepit?'). To apostrophize a character was a favourite device of both Greek and Latin neoteric poets, giving variety and vividness.

**305–6.** The mirror and the constant rearranging of her hair derives from Venus' toilet before the Judgement of Paris in Callimachus, *hymn* 5. 21–2 Κύπρις δὲ διαυγέα χαλκὸν ἑλοῖσα / πολλάκι τὰν αὐτὰν δὶς μετέθηκε κόμαν (cf. Tibullus i. 8. 10 'saepeque mutatas disposuisse comas'). Earlier poets may have exploited the comic possibilities of Pasiphae's failure to interest the bull by orthodox means; compare Propertius iii. 19. 11–12 'testis Cretaei fastus quae passa iuuenci / induit abiegnae cornua falsa bouis.'

**307. crede tamen speculo :** If you *must* take a mirror with you, then at least accept its verdict (cf. Martial ii. 41. 8 'quare si speculo mĭhique credis').

**308. quam cuperes fronti cornua nata tuae !** : probably inspired by *Ecl.* 6. 51 'et saepe in leui quaesisset cornua fronte'. 'Nata' is the *vox propria*, as in Horace, *Odes* ii. 20. 11–12 'nascunturque leues / per digitos umerosque plumae.'

**310. uirum . . . uiro** : playing on the double sense of *uir* (first 'husband', then 'man'). Eleanor Leach (*TAPA* 1964, 143 n. 1[a]) refers to Euripides' *Cretans* (Page, Loeb *Gk. Lit. Pap.* p. 74 lines 6–8) where Pasiphae argues that she would justly have been condemned had she preferred another *man* to her husband; as things are, her passion must be divinely inspired!

**311-12.** Such pictures of women distraught with love or grief are frequent (e.g. *Aen.* iv. 68 ff., vii. 376–7, Propertius iv. 4. 71–2, [Virgil], *Ciris* 165 ff.), in this case perhaps owing something to the sick imaginings of Phaedra (Euripides, *Hippolytus* 215 ff.). Equally conventional is the comparison with a Maenad (see Pease on *Aeneid* iv. 301).

**312. Aonio**: 'Boeotian'—Bacchus' mother was the Theban princess Semele.

**313 ff.** Pasiphae's treatment of any good-looking cow exactly parallels some cruel queen in Tragedy punishing a rival who had won her royal husband's affection—e.g. the myth of Dirce and Antiope (Propertius iii. 15), on which Euripides and Pacuvius had written famous plays. Compare particularly Propertius iii. 15. 13–18:

> a quotiens pulchros uulsit regina capillos,
> molliaque immitis fixit in ora manus!
> a quotiens famulam pensis onerauit iniquis,
> et caput in dura ponere iussit humo!
> saepe illam immundis passa est habitare tenebris,
> uilem ieiunae saepe negauit aquam.

**313. a, quotiens** (or sometimes 'o, quotiens') belongs mainly to the sentimental neoteric and elegiac style. Often the phrase is repeated, as in the Tibullus and Propertius lines quoted on 299–300 and 313 ff. (see further Shackleton Bailey, *Propertiana*, pp. 304–5).

**314. domino . . . meo** : The endearment (cf. *Amores* iii. 7. 11 'et mihi blanditias dixit, dominumque uocauit') is in this context intentionally grotesque.

**316.** 'And the silly creature probably thinks that it becomes her!'

**317. iamdudum** : 'immediately', perhaps with the implication that she had long wished to do so (cf. Austin on *Aeneid* ii. 103 'iamdudum sumite poenas').

**319. commentaque sacra** : 'and an invented ceremony'. By itself 'cadere ante sacra' would be most peculiar Latin, but the association with 'aras' just about saves it. For the use of religion in love's interest cf. Propertius iv. 4. 23–4 (Tarpeia) 'saepe illa immeritae causata est omina lunae / et sibi tingendas dixit in amne comas.'

**321–2.** The climax, with some repetition of words for emphasis. This should not make us suspect the couplet; if anything we could better omit 319–20, thus bringing 'quotiens' (321) into relation with 'a quotiens' (313).

**321. placauit numina :** a grandiose phrase (cf. Cicero, fr. 22. 9 Morel 'aurigeris diuom placantes numina tauris') adding irony —as if Pasiphae's indulgence of her morbid jealousy could win divine approval!

**322. 'ite, placete meo' :** 'Go on, please my beloved', i.e. 'this is what happens to those who please my beloved.' 'Meus' ('mea') alone is lover's language like 'dominus' (314).

**323.** Europa was carried away by Zeus in the form of a bull, while Io was herself changed into a cow, either by Zeus to conceal his love-affair with her, or by Hera in jealousy.
For the elision of the monosyllable *se* (recurring at 327) cf. Platnauer, *Latin Elegiac Verse*, pp. 76 ff. He notes the relative frequency with which m(e), t(e) and s(e) are cut off.

**325–6.** Daedalus made for Pasiphae a counterfeit cow, so that she gained her desire, and bore the Minotaur.

**326. et partu proditus auctor erat :** cf. *Met.* viii. 155–6 'foedumque patebat / matris adulterium monstri nouitate biformis' (with my note for possible echoes of Euripides' *Cretans*).

**327 ff.** Euripidean Tragedy was much in Ovid's mind round about here. He had just finished with the subject-matter of the *Cretans* (Pasiphae). 335–6 remind us of the *Medea*; also lurking in the background are three other plays with notoriously shameless heroines, the *Cretan Women* (cf. 327–30), the *Phoenix* (cf. 337), and the earlier *Hippolytus* (cf. 338).

**327–30.** Aerope ('the Cretan woman', 327), wife of Atreus, fell in love with her brother-in-law Thyestes, setting in motion the events culminating in the banquet at which Thyestes unwittingly ate his own children, making the sun turn back in horror.

**327. Cressa :** The previous heroine, Pasiphae, had also come from Crete; readers would be helped in switching their thoughts by the title of Euripides' Κρῆσσαι (*Cretan Women*) in which Aerope was the protagonist (see T. B. L. Webster, *The Tragedies of Euripides* (1967), pp. 37–9). Numerous other plays on the same legend are catalogued by S. G. Owen on *Tristia* ii. 391; most recent would be the *Thyestes* of Varius, glory of the Roman stage.

**328.** 'And what a great matter it is, to be able to manage without one particular man!' This interpretation of R. Pichon, supported by Kenney, gives good sense. 'Quantum' is ironic, i.e. Ovid really means that it was not much to ask of Aerope that she should keep away from her brother-in-law. Perhaps, however, we should punctuate the line as a question with E. Courtney, who compares *Met.* iv. 74–5, ix. 561. ' Posse carere' seems colloquial and sarcastic, cf. Martial iii. 53, ending 'tota te poteram, Chloe, carere.'

**329–30.** For the sun turning back we can quote a fine fragment of Accius' *Atreus* (183–5 Warmington) 'sed quid tonitru turbida toruo / concussa repente aequora caeli / sensimus sonere?'

**331–2.** Ovid here identifies two heroines normally separated (they both appear in the *Metamorphoses*): (a) Scylla daughter of Nisus, who fell in love with Minos when he was besieging Megara, and betrayed the city to him by cutting off her father's magic lock; she was eventually transformed into a bird (cf. *Met.* viii. 6–151) and (b) Scylla who became a sea-monster (cf. *Met.* xiii. 898 ff.). Of course a poet need not always follow the same version of a legend, and the identification had been made before (see my note on *Met.* viii. 121). Almost all manuscripts here carry two spurious lines, clumsily inserted between 331 and 332 to keep the heroines distinct. An unknown tragedian, perhaps a follower of Euripides, had written on Scylla daughter of Nisus (cf. *Tristia* ii. 393–4), but we cannot tell what form of the legend he adopted.

**332** = *Amores* iii. 12. 22. For the description of the sea-monster cf. Lucretius v. 892–3 'rabidis canibus succinctas semimarinis / corporibus Scyllas', imitated by Virgil at *Ecl.* 6. 75.

**333–4.** Agamemnon escaped two hostile gods in their own element, but fell victim to his wife Clytemnestra at home, as he himself tells Odysseus in the underworld (*Od.* xi. 406–11):

> οὔτ' ἐμέ γ' ἐν νήεσσι Ποσειδάων ἐδάμασσεν
> ὅρσας ἀργαλέων ἀνέμων ἀμέγαρτον ἀϋτμήν,
> οὔτε μ' ἀνάρσιοι ἄνδρες ἐδηλήσαντ' ἐπὶ χέρσου,
> ἀλλά μοι Αἴγισθος τεύξας θάνατόν τε μόρον τε
> ἔκτα σὺν οὐλομένῃ ἀλόχῳ, οἶκόνδε καλέσσας
> δειπνίσσας, ὥς τίς τε κατέκτανε βοῦν ἐπὶ φάτνῃ.

('Neither did Poseidon cause my downfall on ship-board by raising a horrible blast of unfavourable winds, nor did hostile men do me harm on the land, but Aegisthus devised death and destruction for me, and killed me with the help of my cursed wife, after inviting me home and entertaining me, as one slaughters an ox in the stall.')

**333. Martem :** warfare in general, but also alluding to *Iliad* v where the god comes down to fight for the Trojans.

**terra :** cf. ἐπὶ χέρσου in *Od.* xi. 408 (above) just as 'in undis' corresponds to ἐν νήεσσι (406).

**Neptunum effugit in undis :** particularly the violent storm which wrecked the Greek fleet on the way back from Troy (cf. Aeschylus, *Agamemnon* 650 ff.).

**334. uictima dira :** a much more vivid metaphor than 'victim' for us. No doubt Ovid has in mind Homer's comparison of Agamemnon to a slaughtered ox (*Od.* xi. 411 above). Also 'dirus' is often used in the sphere of divination; the murder of Agamemnon was a sacrifice that boded ill for his wife.

**335–6.** Creusa was the Corinthian ('Ephyraean') princess whom Jason married after setting aside Medea. The last-named murdered her rival by means of a poisoned robe, and then killed her own children. Ovid seems to imply that Creusa and Medea were equally culpable.

**335. cui non defleta est :** 'What poet has not told the sad story of . . . ?' Compare Virgil, *Georgics* iii. 6 'cui non dictus Hylas puer?', [Virgil], *Aetna* 21 'quis non periurae doluit mendacia puppis?' There may be a small joke at his own expense—not so long ago Ovid himself had written a tragedy on Medea which later generations valued highly (Quintilian x. 1. 98, cf. Tacitus, *Dialogus* 12).

   **flamma :** in two senses, both her 'passion' and her 'burning', since the poisoned robe burst into flames when put on (cf. Horace, *Epode* 5. 65–6 'cum palla, tabo munus imbutum, nouam / incendio nuptam abstulit'). Propertius has the same *double entendre* at ii. 16. 30 'arserit et quantis nupta Creusa malis'.

**336.** Cf. *Eclogues* 8. 47–8 'saeuus Amor docuit natorum sanguine matrem / commaculare manus.'

**337 ff.** We end with three stories of the Potiphar's wife type, which show innocent men being ruined by women's passion. First, Amyntor believed the slanders of his mistress Pthia against his son Phoenix, and blinded him, a myth treated in Euripides' lost *Phoenix* (see Webster, *The Tragedies of Euripides*, pp. 84–5).

**337. inania lumina :** cf. Valerius Flaccus iv. 435 'oculos attollit inanes.' This use of *inanis* for *caecus* may be suggested by Ap. Rh. ii. 254–5 κενεὰς ὁ γεραιὸς ἀνέσχε / γλήνας ἀμπετάσας and ibid. 445 (cited by Kenney (*CR* 1966, 270–1), who also disposes of Housman's clever but misguided conjecture 'lucis' for 'Phoenix' at the end of the line). Note Lycophron, *Al.* 422 on Phoenix.

**338. Hippolytum rabidi diripuistis equi :** Falsely accused by his step-mother Phaedra, Hippolytus was cursed by his father Theseus and driven into exile. In answer to the curse Poseidon sent a bull from the sea which threw the horses into confusion, so causing fatal injuries to Hippolytus. This forms the subject of one of the finest and most influential Euripidean tragedies; we should remember that in the lost earlier *Hippolytus* Phaedra's conduct was much more shameless, drawing severe criticism on to the playwright (see W. S. Barrett's *Hippolytus*, pp. 10–45, Webster, *Tragedies of Euripides*, pp. 64 ff.).

In this line, as often elsewhere, we must choose between the variants 'rabidi' and 'pauidi'. Either can be supported from Euripides (*Hipp.* 1230 and 1218 respectively). Like Kenney I rather prefer 'rabidi', mainly because it combines more force-fully with 'diripuistis'; for the other view see Goold, *Harvard Studies* 69 (1965), 63.

**339–40.** Curiously linked to 337 by the theme of blinding (this punishment for a sexual crime is discussed by G. Devereux in a strange article (*JHS* 1973, 40 ff.)). The story is almost identical; for the varying names of Phineus' sons and his second wife, see Frazer on Apollodorus iii. 15. 3, and ibid. i. 9. 21 for the later blinding of Phineus. Both Aeschylus and Sophocles composed tragedies on Phineus.

**341–4.** Ending of the section, linked to 281–2 and 269–70.

**343. ergo age :** drawing the lesson from previous examples, as at *Georgics* i. 63 (Kenney in *Ovidiana*, p. 203).

**345–50.** *Postscript: even if you fail, no harm will be done. But why should you fail?*

**346. ut iam fallaris:** 'even supposing, then, you are disappointed . . .'.

**347. cum sit noua grata uoluptas :** 'Variety is the spice of life', or as the Greeks put it μεταβολὴ πάντων γλυκύ (see Otto, *Sprich-wörter*, s.v. Varietas).

**348–50.** Three proverbs of the type 'The grass is always greener . . .'. See Otto, s.v. Alienus 1; particularly close parallels are respectively (a) Publilius Syrus 28 'aliena nobis, nostra plus aliis placent', (b) Juvenal 14. 142–3 'maiorque uidetur / et melior uicina seges' and (c) Horace, *Sat.* i. 1. 110 'aliena capella gerat distentius uber'.

**351–98.** *Before making a move, you should get to know the girl's maid* (the second of three preliminary sections (see on 269–350)).

The *ancilla* is a familiar figure of Latin love-elegy; two pairs of poems in the *Amores* illustrate her. *Amores* i. 11 and i. 12 concern Nape, who is first sent to Corinna with a message inscribed on a wax tablet; in the second poem Ovid bewails that the answer has come back 'impossible today' (compare 383 here, which refers to the exchange of messages through the maid). *Amores* ii. 7 and ii. 8, the other pair, are notable examples of Ovid's early desire to shock his readers; they cannot be taken as strictly auto-biographical, or else he would hardly have revealed the story! The first piece, addressed to Corinna, is full of injured innocence ('How could you possibly suspect me of having an affair with

your maid Cypassis? The idea is ridiculous—apart from any-
thing else, I'd have gone higher in the social scale') while the
second addresses Cypassis ('How did Corinna learn of our affair?
Did I blush, or make some slip of the tongue? Now you must
grant everything I ask, or else I'll tell all to your mistress').
These poems act as a commentary on the soberly worded dis-
cussion starting at 375.

We can follow the background further; bribing the maid to
get at the mistress is a motif which occurs in Comedy (Plautus,
*Asinaria* 183 ff., cf. *Menaechmi* 540 ff.). The *ancilla* also owes
something to an older character, the Euripidean nurse who acts
as a go-between for the heroine to the man she loves. One
thinks of Phaedra's nurse in the *Hippolytus*, and there must
have been similar parts in tragedies which have not survived.
Finally, in 371–2 the *ancilla* recommends the young man to her
mistress, saying that he is madly in love with her. In this she
performs the office of a much less appetizing person, the *lena*,
who descends to love-elegy through New Comedy and Mime (cf.
372 n.). *Amores* i. 8 concerns such a woman, who opens her
attack on the girl with 'scis here te, mea lux, iuueni placuisse
beato?' (23). This case is fairly typical in that we see various
strands of love-elegy descending from different literary ante-
cedents. Of course one is not denying that such characters and
incidents belonged to contemporary Roman life, but the actual
mode of description is often highly conventional.

**351. captandae . . . puellae :** The attempt on her has not yet begun,
so this Renaissance correction of the manuscripts' 'captatae'
seems necessary (see Kenney in *CQ* 1959, 248–9 against an earlier
note by Alan Ker).

**353–4.** i.e. there is no point in wasting your efforts on a maid who
does not enjoy the close confidence of her mistress. It emerges
from 367 that Ovid is thinking of the *ornatrix*, who as a 'hair
artiste' might be considered a cut above the ordinary maids; cf.
*Amores* i. 11. 1–2 'colligere incertos et in ordine ponere crines /
docta neque ancillas inter habenda Nape', ii. 7. 17–18, ii. 8. 1–2.

**354. parum :** with 'conscia fida' (for a similar hyberbaton involv-
ing 'nimis' see R. G. M. Nisbet on Cicero, *in Pisonem* 17).

**356. ex facili :** 'easily', cf. Tacitus, *Agricola* 15 'tamquam ex
facili tolerantibus'.

**357. (medici quoque tempora seruant) :** just as doctors wait for
precisely the right moment to apply their medicine. The paren-
thesis may seem to have no very good point but it briefly
anticipates the section starting at 399, and, as with the analogies
from hunting etc., we are probably meant to recall that medicine
too was treated in ancient didactic poems—a surviving Latin
example is the *Liber Medicinalis* of Q. Serenus Sammonicus.

**359-74.** *The best times for the maid to approach your intended are when she is happy* (359-64) *or when she is jealous* (365-74).

**359. laetissima rerum :** either 'happiest in the world' (cf. 213) or, as Kenney favours, 'most pleased with life' ('rerum' in that case being an objective genitive, as at *Aeneid* xi. 72 'laeta laborum').

**359-60.** Editors who print no comma at the end of 359 must take 'mens', or even the lady herself, to be subject of 'luxuriabit' (i.e. cum laetissima rerum luxuriabit ut seges in pingui humo). While the verb can well denote mental exuberance (e.g. ii. 437, Livy i. 19), I feel that a comma (understanding 'est' with 'laetissima rerum') gives more force to the comparison. For then the *seges* can represent the maid's suggestion, and the *pinguis humus* the girl's *laeta mens* in which it flourishes (*laetus* is often used of fertile soil, e.g. Varro, *de Re Rustica* i. 23. 7 quoting the elder Cato, 'ager . . . laetus').

**361. adstricta :** literally 'drawn tight', as if by a confining bond, so making a contrast with 'patent' (362).

**363. cum tristis erat :** particularly after the death of Hector. The removal of her greatest champion did not cause Troy's downfall, instead making her defenders all the more alert.

**364. militibus grauidum . . . equum :** The image of the Wooden Horse as pregnant with Greek warriors goes back to Ennius, *Alexander* 80-1 Warmington 'grauidus armatis equus / qui suo partu ardua perdat Pergama'. It was taken up notably by Lucretius and Virgil (see Austin on *Aeneid* ii. 237), but Ovid knew Ennius well and (as the close verbal resemblance suggests) probably draws direct from the old poet.

　　**laeta :** Readers would call to mind *Aeneid* ii. 26 ff. (after the supposed departure of the Greeks) 'ergo omnis longo soluit se Teucria luctu: / panduntur portae etc.' and ibid. 237-9 'scandit fatalis machina muros / feta armis. pueri circum innuptaeque puellae / sacra canunt funemque manu contingere gaudent.'

**365. cum paelice laesa dolebit :** like the girl-friend's *uir*, a vestigial trace of a situation in which she is thought of as a married woman, although Ovid more than once insists that he is writing only for *hetaerae*. See further Introduction pp. xvi-xvii.

**368. uelo remigis addat opem :** proverbial for hastening something on by all possible means, e.g. Plautus, *Asin.* 157 'remigio ueloque quantum poteris festina et fuge' (Otto, *Sprichwörter*, s.v. Remus).

**369. tenui . . . murmure :** cf. Juvenal 4. 110 of a whispering campaign 'tenui iugulos aperire susurro'.

**370.** 'But, I suppose, you couldn't pay him back in his own coin.' The imperfect 'poteras' implies a tentative suggestion (as e.g. at *Met.* i. 679, viii. 47); coupled with Burman's conjecture 'at' this gives very much more pointed sense than 'ut puto, . . . poteris'.

**372. et insano iuret amore mori :** We can parallel this situation closely from Hellenistic Mime (see on 351–98). In Herodas 1, Gyllis, after commenting on the long absence and probable infidelity of Metriche's husband in Egypt, mentions the young man Gryllus (48 ff.) adding καί μευ οὔτε νυκτὸς οὔτ' ἐπ' ἡμέρην λείπει / τὸ δῶμα, τέκνον, ἀλλά μευ κατακλαίει / καὶ ταταλίζει καὶ ποθέων ἀποθνῄσκει (58–60, 'and, child, he does not leave my house by night or day, but weeps before me, coaxes me and is dying of love').

**373. uela . . . auraeque :** continuing the metaphor of 368.

**375–98.** *Should you try to enjoy the favours of the maid herself? Such a course is hardly to be recommended.* Compare the two poems on Cypassis (*Amores* ii. 7 and 8) mentioned on 351–98. In the present passage Ovid's language becomes more measured and sober (particularly 380, 381, 387–8) as his subject-matter becomes more provocative.

**375. quaeris an . . . ? :** For the didactic question Kenney (in *Ovidiana*, p. 203) cites *Georgics* ii. 288 'forsitan et scrobibus quae sint fastigia quaeras' (add e.g. Manilius iii. 203).

**376. talibus admissis alea grandis inest :** Both here and in 381 'non ego per praeceps et acuta cacumina uadam' Ovid has in mind an epigram probably by Philodemus (*Anth. Pal.* v. 25 = Gow–Page, *The Garland of Philip*, Philodemus no. 3) which contains the same images: when indulging in a dangerous love οἶδ' ὅτι πὰρ κρημνὸν τέμνω πόρον, οἶδ' ὅτι ῥιπτῶ / πάντα κύβον κεφαλῆς αἰὲν ὕπερθεν ἐμῆς (lines 3–4 'I know I am cutting a path beside a precipice, I know I am tossing all the dice overhead each time'). Philodemus himself lived and worked in Italy for a considerable time and had great influence on Roman writers of the late Republic and early Empire (cf. R. G. M. Nisbet's edition of Cicero, *in Pisonem*, Appendix III).

**379. casus in euentu est :** 'The proof of this gamble lies in its outcome'; *casus* (literally 'fall of the dice' as at Juvenal 1. 90) continues the figure of 376. For different forms of the proverb, see Otto, *Sprichwörter*, s.v. Euentus; Ovid elsewhere puts it concisely, 'exitus acta probat' (*Heroides* 2. 85).

**380.** 'Ovide discute les questions douteuses comme un juriste dissertait sur une espèce contestée du droit civil' (R. Pichon).

**381.** See on 376.

**383. dum dat recipitque tabellas :** A long correspondence between the young man and the girl is envisaged (437 ff.).

**387. si quid modo creditur arti :** 'if you have even the slightest confidence in my instruction'. 'Ars' here = the laying down of rules for the subject ('praeceptio quae dat certam uiam rationemque dicendi', *Rhetorica ad Herennium* i. 3).

**388.** For having one's words blown over the sea cf. Theocritus 22. 167–8 ἴσκον τοιάδε πολλά, τὰ δ᾽ εἰς ὑγρὸν ᾤχετο κῦμα / πνοιῇ ἔχουσ᾽ ἀνέμοιο (more in Otto, s.v. Ventus 2, Nisbet and Hubbard on Horace, *Odes* i. 26. 2). Ovid is particularly fond of the figure.

**389.** aut †non temptasses† : The general sense is clear—'either finish the job properly or don't start'—what we should read less so. Heinsius's 'aut non temptaris' (essentially the reading of B) remains perhaps the most plausible try. Note that we would then have a rare example of *non* for *ne* with the perfect subjunctive in a prohibition; scholars compare Catullus 66. 91 'non siris', though 'siris' is in origin an optative form (see Fordyce ad loc.). Quintilian (i. 5. 50) censures the use of 'non feceris' for 'ne feceris' in a prohibition, perhaps implying that it was a current, though mistaken, idiom in his own day. Other more recent attempts to mend our passage are 'aut nolim temptes' (Lenz, *Opuscula Selecta*, pp. 495–6) and 'aut non rem temptes' (Courtney, *CR* 1970, 10).

Professor Nisbet wonders whether one might conceivably retain 'aut non temptasses', translating 'Either you should not have made an attempt on her or finish the job properly' (with the two propositions on different levels as a humorous touch). A pluperfect subjunctive of past obligation causes no difficulty, e.g. *Aeneid* iv. 678 'eadem me ad fata uocasses.' One problem is that we would expect 'ne' rather than 'non' as at Cicero, *ad Att.* ii. 1. 3 'ne poposcisses' (note, however, Plautus, *Trinummus* 133 'non redderes').

**389–90.** Compare Juvenal 6, Oxford fragment 33 'crimen commune tacetur.'

**391–3.** Two facts about these lines seem inescapable to me: (a) they must all make the same point (for the threefold analogy from fowling, hunting, and fishing see on 45–8), (b) they must reinforce the message of 389 and 394, 'either don't make the attempt or finish the job properly'. Therefore Ovid is surely saying that for a fowler, hunter, or fisherman to do his work half-heartedly and let the creature escape is most inglorious.

As far as I can judge from some unusually evasive translations, most scholars take the liming of the bird's wings and the setting of the nets as equivalent to enjoying the maid's favours. Accordingly they interpret 'non . . . utiliter' (391) and 'non bene' (392) as meaning that the creatures are unable to escape. But it is not enough merely to lay your trap; the whole operation must be carried out thoroughly and efficiently (cf. Rhianus, *Anth. Pal.* xii. 146, on the man who set up his nets but lost his love to another).

**391.** 'It is not profitable when a bird flies away after its wings have been smeared with lime.' For the operation correctly performed

contrast Valerius Flaccus, *Argonautica* vi. 260–4 'qualem popu-
leae fidentem nexibus umbrae / si quis auem summi deducat
ab aere rami / ante manu tacita cui plurima creuit harundo; /
illa dolis uiscoque super correpta sequaci / implorat ramos atque
inrita concitat alas.'

    **non . . . utiliter:** For the reasons explained above he can hardly
mean either that the bird is unable to escape, or that, even if it
can, there is no advantage in doing so. 'Non . . . utiliter' then
must be from the fowler's point of view, like 'non bene' in 392
(cf. *Heroides* i. 67, *Tristia* v. 7. 38).

**392.** 'It is disgraceful when a boar makes its way out of the
bulging net.' Ovid seems to envisage a funnel-net with a pro-
nounced belly or pocket (cf. Xenophon, *Cynegeticus* 6. 7, 10. 7);
the epithet 'laxis' (not, I think, intended to explain the hunter's
failure) refers to this bulging shape. The hunter shows incom-
petence by neglecting to close the entrance of the net, so that
the boar is able to escape back through the opening by which
he came in (cf. 'exit').

    **non bene:** cf. 180 'signaque barbaricas non bene (a reproach
to Romans) passa manus'.

**393.** The emphasis falls on 'teneatur': once a fish has seized the
bait it is up to the fisherman not to let it get off the hook.

**395–6.** These lines are omitted by two important manuscripts,
and Merkel was almost certainly right to delete them. While
Latinity and metre do not give great cause for complaint
(although 396 is feeble), their sentiments are exactly the same
as 389–90 and 398 respectively.

**397. celetur:** probably an impersonal passive.

**398.** 'Your girl will always be subject to your knowledge.'

**399–436.** *You must realize that some times are much better than
others for making a start. Avoid any occasion when you will be
expected to bring a present, and only move when the shops are shut.
But, however many precautions you take, you are certain to have to
pay out in the end.*

    This last preliminary section before Ovid finally tells us how
to start the affair (437 ff.) is one of the most entertaining
passages in the whole work, vivid in its description of Roman
social life and richly complex in combining didactic elements
with those from love-epigram and elegy. Note first of all that the
section is based on the 'Days' of Hesiod's *Works and Days*
(lines 765–828) wherein the poet lays down which days are
favourable and which unfavourable for specific tasks (cf. Virgil,
*Georgics* i. 276 ff.).

**399–400.** 'The man who thinks that only farmers and sailors
need observe the seasons is mistaken.' Virgil had said that a

farmer must pay as much attention to the seasons as a sailor (*Georgics* i. 204–7):

> praeterea tam sunt Arcturi sidera nobis
> Haedorumque dies seruandi et lucidus Anguis
> quam quibus in patriam uentosa per aequora uectis
> Pontus et ostriferi fauces temptantur Abydi.

Our poet adds that the lover must be no less observant than either of them.

**400. fallitur :** Kenney compares Lucretius ii. 80–2 'si cessare putas rerum primordia posse / . . . auius a uera longe ratione uagaris.'

Ovid dislocates his sentence by enclosing the main verb 'fallitur' within a relative clause. One can see here a mannerism deriving from the Hellenistic poets, particularly Callimachus (cf. Gordon Williams, *Tradition and Originality in Roman Poetry*, pp. 714–16); for Ovidian hyperbaton see Housman, *JP* 18 (1890), 7, Postgate, *CR* 30 (1916), 142 ff., Platnauer, *Latin Elegiac Verse*, pp. 104 ff., Marouzeau in *Ovidiana*, pp. 101–5. The most violent trajection occurs in a poem commonly thought not to be by Ovid, *Amores* iii. 5. 13–14 'candidior, quod adhuc spumis stridentibus albet / et modo siccatam, lacte, reliquit ouem' ('lacte' is ablative of comparison after 'candidior') but hardly less striking is *Tristia* iii. 9. 12 ' "hospes" ait "nosco Colchide uela uenit" ' (i.e. hospes Colchide uenit—nosco uela).

**401. nec semper credenda Ceres fallacibus aruis :** recalling *Georgics* i. 224, the time must be right before 'inuitae properes anni spem credere terrae'.

**403. nec . . . semper tutum :** suggesting particularly Hesiod's advice on when sailing was safe and when unsafe (*Works and Days* 618–94).

**404. dato . . . tempore :** 'when the correct moment presents itself'.

**melius . . . fiet idem :** 'The same action (as you might perform on a less favourable occasion) will turn out better.' But there may be something idiomatic here which eludes me; elsewhere 'fiet idem' are the words of a procrastinator (*Remedia* 104 'cras quoque fiet idem').

**405. siue dies suberit natalis :** Birthdays were observed with great ceremony at Rome (see Balsdon, *Life and Leisure in Ancient Rome*, pp. 121–2) and particularly the poets in Messalla's circle liked to write birthday elegies (several examples in Tibullus and the *Corpus Tibullianum*, cf. Propertius iii. 10). We hear more about the girl's birthday, real or fictitious, at 417 and 429–30.

**405–6. siue Kalendae, / quas Venerem Marti continuasse iuuat :** 'or those merry Kalends which join Venus' month to that of Mars', briefly recalling Hesiod and Virgil where specific days of the month are favourable or unfavourable (see on 399–436). Surely the first of April must be meant; this month was sacred to the goddess and on the Kalends she received worship both from Roman matrons and those of lower status—'rite deam colitis Latiae matresque nurusque / et uos, quis uittae longaque uestis abest' (*Fasti* iv. 133–4, see Frazer ad loc.). Line 406 probably contains a side allusion to the love-affair of Venus and Mars (cf. *Fasti* iv. 129–30 for the wording).

Some scholars have seen a reference to 1 March, the *Matronalia* (for which cf. Balsdon, *Life and Leisure*, p. 124); this view has the advantage that we know the *Matronalia* to have been an occasion for presents, but it can hardly be squared with the mention of Venus.

**407–8. siue erit ornatus non, ut fuit ante, sigillis, / sed regum positas Circus habebit opes :** 'Or if the Circus (no longer decked out with statuettes as in the old days) has royal treasures on display . . .' Difficult lines. The mention of *sigilla* points to the market called Sigillaria which was linked to the great December festival of the Saturnalia, and provided an occasion for the exchange of gifts, but some details are obscure.

**non, ut fuit ante, sigillis :** If my translation is correct, these words perform two functions, (a) showing that Ovid refers to the Sigillaria, (b) making the point that while former generations were content with clay statuettes (whence the market's name), present tastes are more expensive, and you would have no hope of getting away with such a token gift (see Balsdon, *Life and Leisure*, p. 124). To paraphrase: 'if it is the time of the Sigillaria (but today they sell more costly things than *sigilla*) . . .' For a similar touch cf. ii. 267–8 'quas Amaryllis amabat, / at nunc, castaneas, non amat illa, nuces'. Juvenal 6. 153–7, partly quoted below, describes items of enormous value being bought at the Sigillaria.

Mr. N. J. Richardson suggested the basis of the above interpretation to me. Most people seem to follow Brandt, who concluded that *after* the Sigillaria (i.e. during the New Year celebrations) clay statuettes and other such trinkets were replaced in the market by more expensive items.

**408. regum . . . opes :** probably just objects of great worth, though some might have a notable pedigree, as in Juvenal 6. 155–7 :

> grandia tolluntur crystallina, maxima rursus
> myrrhina, deinde adamas notissimus et Berenices
> in digito factus pretiosior.

**Circus :** presumably the Circus Maximus, since no qualification is added. So it appears that in Ovid's day the market of the Sigillaria was held in the Circus Maximus; in Juvenal's time it was in the Colonnade of the Argonauts, later still in a colonnade of Trajan's Baths (scholiast on Juvenal 6. 154). Possibly, however, the Circus Flaminius might be in question (called simply 'Circus' at *Fasti* vi. 205, 209); Martial (xii. 74. 2) speaks of a cup bought there. See T. P. Wiseman, *Papers of the British School at Rome* 42 (1974), 3–26.

**409. tunc tristis hiems :** perhaps understand *instat*—'then ugly storms and the Pliades threaten.' Alternatively 'that is the time of gloomy winter [like Virgil's 'hiems ignaua colono', *Georgics* i. 299] when the Pliades threaten.' In any case we should put out of our minds the fact that the Sigillaria (and also the setting of the Kids (410)) actually took place in December. Since the lover's sea-faring is purely metaphorical (411–12), the indications of climate are best confined to the same level; they represent the lover's close season and financial dangers for him on the horizon (cf. *Remedia* 739–40 'haec tibi sint Syrtes, haec Acroceraunia uita: / hic uomit epotas dira Charybdis aquas'). Therefore there is no need to observe that courting is 'made even more distasteful by the wet weather usual at the time of year' (M. J. Griggs in his *Selections*).

**Pliades :** for their association with storms cf. Hesiod, *Works and Days* 619, Virgil, *Georgics* iv. 234–5.

**410. tunc tener aequorea mergitur Haedus aqua :** the most notoriously dangerous time for sailing, cf. *Met.* xiv. 711 'saeuior illa freto surgente cadentibus Haedis', Callimachus, *Ep.* 18 Pf. 5–6 (an epitaph) φεῦγε θαλάσσῃ / συμμίσγειν Ἐρίφων, ναυτίλε, δυομένων, Nicaenetus, *Anth. Pal.* vii. 502. 4, Aratus, *Phaen.* 158–9.

**411–12. tunc si quis creditur alto, / uix tenuit lacerae naufraga membra ratis :** i.e. the lover will incur disastrous financial loss.

The lines well illustrate the complexity of the *Ars*. On one level we have a melancholy reflection on the fate of those who go to sea at the wrong time, in the didactic style of Hesiod (*Works and Days* 618 ff.), Aratus and his followers (see on 412), and Virgil (*Georgics* i. 456–7 'non illa quisquam me nocte per altum / ire neque a terra moneat conuellere funem'). On another level we are to recognize a favourite image of love-elegy and epigram: those whom love ruined were said to be 'shipwrecked on the sea of Venus', 'nudus, egens, Veneris naufragus in pelago' as Porfyrius put it (fr. 1 Morel—more material in Nisbet and Hubbard on Horace, *Odes* i. 5. 16) while the man who achieves happiness or escapes unhappiness will come safely to port—'ecce coronatae portum tetigere carinae, / traiectae Syrtes, ancora iacta mea est' (Propertius iii. 24. 15–16, cf. ii. 14. 29–30, Ovid, *A.A.* ii. 9–10).

**412.** 'That man can barely cling to a broken spar of his shattered vessel.' Ovid may echo Cicero's youthful adaptation of Aratus.

Buescu assigned the stray line 'nauibus absumptis fluitantia quaerere aplustra' (fr. 25) to the fate of men who sail when the Kids are setting (cf. 410 above). Although this would represent a considerable expansion of the original (158–9), both Germanicus (*Aratea* 171–3) and Avienus (417–20) also expand at this point. Contrast Hesiod, *Works and Days* 665–6: if you sail at the right time οὔτε κε νῆα / καυάξαις οὔτ' ἄνδρας ἀποφθείσειε θάλασσα ('you are not likely to break up your ship, nor the sea to destroy the crew').

**413–14.** One of the blackest days in the Roman Calendar, 18 July, anniversary of a catastrophic defeat by the Gauls at the river Allia (390 B.C.). Virgil cannot mention the name without a sigh— 'quosque secans infaustum interluit Allia nomen' (*Aeneid* vii. 717). For this and other *dies atri* see Balsdon, *Life and Leisure*, pp. 66 and 370. Public business would cease and the shops close, so that the impecunious lover does not risk having to buy a present. Ovid displays a grim kind of humour in saying that all cheerful festivals are out, but the *dies Alliensis* is excellent!

**413. tum licet :** I somewhat prefer 'tu licet' (in a permissive sense also at Martial viii. 55. 12) which has stronger manuscript support. The pronoun would link up with 'tibi' in 417: *you* (unlike your fellow countrymen) may work on the 'dies Alliensis', but *your* black day (unlike theirs) will be a birthday or any cheerful festival (cf. on 417–18).

**415–16.** Ovid's second reference to Judaism (see on 76 for a fuller note), which obviously had a significant impact on the economic as well as the social life of Rome—an appreciable number of shops would be shut on the Sabbath. He need not refer particularly to Jewish shopkeepers (it does not appear that Roman Jews engaged in commerce more than other occupations); many Gentiles might follow the basic prohibitions of Judaism without embracing that religion in its entirety (cf. Juvenal 14. 96 'metuentem sabbata patrem').

**415. rebus minus apta gerendis :** At *Remedia* 219–20 Ovid shows himself aware of the restriction on Sabbath journeying. Some Romans affected to despise the weekly rest-day, e.g. Rutilius Namatianus i. 391 'septima quaeque dies turpi damnata ueterno' (cf. Seneca *ap.* Augustine, *de Civ. Dei* vi. 11, Tacitus, *Histories* v. 4).

**417–18.** Nicely linked to 413–16 by *superstitio* and *atra dies*. You should feel inhibited not (as one might imagine) on the Jewish Sabbath, but rather on her birthday; your black day is not the *dies Alliensis* (as for your fellow countrymen) but any occasion when a present is due.

**417. magna superstitio :** 'an object of great dread', and therefore something you will take care to avoid, cf. *Aeneid* xii. 817 (the oath by the Styx) 'una superstitio superis quae reddita diuis'. In a similar spirit the *Works and Days* and the *Georgics* warn against especially ill-omened days.

**419–20.** For an attack upon love because it wastes one's property cf. Lucretius iv. 1121 ff.

**420. carpat** : 'fleece', a metaphor from sheep-shearing and slightly colloquial (although the verb does not seem to occur in the literal sense of 'tondere'). Propertius' advice to Cynthia con-concerning his rich rival was 'stolidum pleno uellere carpe pecus' (ii. 16. 8, cf. Ovid, *Amores* i. 8. 91 and Headlam on Herodas 3. 39 for the similar use of κείρω).

**421–8.** *The door-to-door salesman*, a lively vignette which seems to breathe the atmosphere of Comedy and Mime. I do not know any very close parallel, but see Headlam's Introduction to his *Herodas*, pp. xlvii–li on Mimes 6 and 7 ('The Cobbler').

**421. institor** : He had a bad reputation, as shown by Horace, *Epode* 17. 20 'amata nautis multum et institoribus', cf. *Odes* iii. 6. 30 (quoted on 565 ff.), Ovid, *Remedia* 306.

  **discinctus** : 'loose'. The word means literally 'wearing no belt with his tunic', and this was the typical dress of an *institor* (Propertius iv. 2. 38 'mundus demissis institor in tunicis'); the Roman working classes would normally wear a tunic without a toga above it (cf. Gudeman on Tacitus, *Dialogus* 7. 4 'tunicatus hic populus', Lillian M. Wilson, *The Clothing of the Ancient Romans*, pp. 55 ff.). But since in ancient more than modern times irregularity of dress was thought to indicate moral or political irregularity—note Sulla's warning against the young Julius Caesar 'ut male praecinctum puerum cauerent' (Suetonius, *Diuus Julius* 45)—'discinctus' had connotations of moral laxity which fit the *institor*'s ill repute (above).

  **emacem** : 'bargain-hungry'.

**423. sapere ut uideare** : 'so that you give the impression of being a connoisseur'.

**426. bene . . . emi** : 'it is cheap at the price', like the French *bon marché*. Compare Quintilian, *Decl.* 253 'bene . . . redimi capite unius ciuis pacem', and contrast Plautus, *Amphitruo* 288 'conducto male' of something over-priced (also *Amores* i. 10. 44).

**427. causabere** : 'you plead in excuse'.

  **nummos** : 'cash', somewhat colloquial as at Horace, *Epist.* i. 1. 54 'uirtus post nummos'. The same applies to 'domi', 'on you', 'readily available', cf. e.g. Martial vii. 16. 1 'aera domi non sunt.'

**428. littera poscetur** : 'you will be asked for your signature' (on a note promising to pay later). The essence of 'littera' here is a personal and identifiable hand, 'something in writing', as at Juvenal 13. 138 'arguit ipsorum quos littera'.

**ne didicisse iuuet :** 'just to make you wish you were illiterate'.
The formally final clause adds a touch of irony which should not
be obscured by saying that ne = ut non (see R. G. Nisbet *AJP*
44 (1923), 27–43). For the sentiment compare Nero's reported
words when asked to sign a death-warrant, 'uellem litteras
nescirem' (Seneca, *de Clem.* ii. 1). Here we can either supply
'litteras' from the singular 'littera' preceding or (as I would
prefer) understand 'didicisse' absolutely; a similar case is
*Tristia* ii. 343–4 'heu mihi quod didici, quod me docuere paren-
tes, / litteraque est oculos ulla morata meos.'

**429–30.** 'What of the times when she demands a gift by pro-
ducing a supposed birthday-cake, and has a lucrative birthday
as often as the need arises?'

**429. quasi natali . . . libo :** ablative, 'with a supposed birthday-
cake' (not dative, 'as if to buy a birthday-cake'), as indicated
by *Amores* i. 8. 94 'natalem libo testificare tuum'. For the
addition of *quasi* cf. Pliny, *Epist.* viii. 16. 1 'quasi testamenta',
Tacitus, *Ann.* xii. 41 'his quasi criminibus'.

**430. et, quotiens opus est, nascitur illa sibi :** Many translators
understand the line simply as = nascitur quotiens sibi opus est.
But I feel sure that there is more in it, and that 'nascitur illa
sibi' alludes to Plato's dictum that each man was not born for
himself alone (*Epist.* 9. 358a, cf. Cicero, *de Finibus* ii. 45 'non
sibi se soli natum meminerit, sed patriae, sed suis'). This young
lady, on the other hand, is born for herself, and repeatedly
('nascitur' here carries the double implication 'is born' and
'has a birthday'). It is difficult to convey the sharpness of the
joke in English.

**431–2.** Imaginary losses, which must be replaced at the lover's
expense. Compare Horace, *Epist.* i. 17. 55–6, the importunate
client 'nota refert meretricis acumina, saepe catellam / saepe
periscelidem raptam sibi flentis.' In Plautus' *Truculentus*
(52 ff.) Diniarchus embarks on an unending catalogue of items
which the lover must make good: 'aut periit aurum aut con-
scissa pallula est / aut empta ancilla aut aliquod uasum argen-
teum / aut uasum ahenum etc.' (cf. also Martial xi. 49).

**432. caua :** 'pierced'. For Roman ear-rings, with some illustra-
tion, see Lillian Wilson, *The Clothing of the Ancient Romans*,
pp. 34–5.

**433–4.** On borrowing things which will never be returned cf. the
*lena*'s advice to a girl at *Amores* i. 8. 102 'quod numquam reddas
commodet ipsa roga.' You never see your property again, and
do not even get the gratitude which an outright gift would earn.
Verres tried the same trick: 'primo ille suo leniore artificio
Heraclium aggredi conatur, ut eum roget inspicienda quae non
reddat' (Cicero, *in Verrem* ii. 36).

**435–6. non mihi, sacrilegas meretricum ut persequar artes, / cum totidem linguis sint satis ora decem :** The formula about ten tongues and ten mouths started with Homer (*Iliad* ii. 488–90) and had a long history in serious Latin verse (see my note on *Met.* viii. 533–4); of course its employment for the present context produces intentional bathos. No doubt Ovid would point to *Georgics* ii. 42–4; if in one didactic poem, why not in another?

**437 ff.** Finally the poet reveals how to start winning a young woman—you must write to her, as the first shot in a long campaign. Instructions are given on the content (439–54) and style (459–68) of your letter. Lovers' correspondence plays quite a part in the amatory tradition; see Plautus, *Pseudolus* 20 ff., *Asinaria* 761 ff., Ovid, *Amores* i. 11 and 12, and for the transference of such a scene to higher-style poetry, *Met.* ix. 518 ff. (Byblis). There was even a distinct genre of imaginary love-letters which we see reflected in Ovid's *Heroides* and e.g. the later Greek prose of Aristaenetus.

**437. cera uadum temptet :** reinforcing the nautical imagery prominent of late (399–402, 409–12). The tablet is like a ship on a dangerous journey carrying as cargo ('ferat', 439) the lover's blandishments.

**rasis infusa tabellis :** see E. M. Thompson, *Greek and Latin Palaeography* (1893), pp. 19 ff. for details of ancient writing tablets. A rectangle of wood had a smaller rectangle hollowed out of it on one side, and this was partly filled in with wax, the raised margin which remained round the wax surface preventing rubbing of the wax surface when one tablet was closed against another. In the house of L. Caecilius Jucundus at Pompeii was found a box containing 127 financial tablets (Thompson pp. 24–5). Love-letters apparently might be written on very small tablets which Martial calls 'Vitelliani' (xiv. 8 and 9).

**rasis :** perhaps significant. At iii. 495–6 Ovid warns that one must take care to erase the previous message on a wax tablet—else it may still be readable, with disastrous results!

**438. conscia :** The tablet also plays the part of a go-between, who is often useful in a love-affair (cf. iii. 621, 625, 649, *Amores* i. 11).

**439–40. imitataque amantum / uerba :** an awkward phrase—presumably one must take 'imitata' in a passive sense, 'the imitated words of lovers'. But, with Goold (*Harvard Studies* 69 (1965), 64–5) I prefer the conjecture of Heinsius and Bentley 'amant*em*', 'words which play the lover'. Note the typical uncertainty whether the young man is really in love or just acting a part (cf. 611).

**440. nec exiguas** = et adde non exiguas preces.

**quisquis es :** i.e. however superior you consider yourself.

**441.** Achilles was moved by Priam's entreaties to return the body of Hector (the story from *Iliad* xxiv). For the grandiose *exemplum* in a trivial context cf. Horace, *Epode* 17. 11 ff.

**443. promittas facito :** Ovid gives women an antidote to this at iii. 461 'si bene promittent, totidem promittite uerbis.'

**446.** Poetic accounts of Hope as a goddess spring from Hesiod, *Works and Days* 96 ff.; notable passages are Theognis i. 1135 ff. and Ovid, *ex Ponto* i. 6. 29 ff. (see further K. F. Smith on Tibullus ii. 6. 19–28). For Spes in Roman cult see Nisbet and Hubbard on Horace, *Odes* i. 35. 21, Pease on Cicero, *de Natura Deorum* iii. 47.

**448. praeteritum tulerit perdideritque nihil :** 'She will have gained what is past (i.e. the present you have already given her) and lost nothing (which she might have got by staying with you longer).'

**450. saepe fefellit :** The same field gets repeated chances to prove itself.

**451. ne perdiderit, non cessat perdere lusor :** He goes on losing so as not to be in a state of having lost—a clever word-play. Gambling was traditionally frowned upon in Rome, and even banned by law (see Owen on *Tristia* ii. 472), but the emperor Augustus had a weakness for it which is the subject of an epigram in Suetonius, *Div. Aug.* 70: 'postquam bis classe uictus naues perdidit / aliquando ut uincat ludit assidue aleam.'

**453. hoc opus, hic labor est, primo sine munere iungi :** a notorious line. One can hardly believe that the echo of *Aeneid* vi. 129 is unconscious:

> facilis descensus Auerno:
> noctes atque dies patet atri ianua Ditis;
> sed reuocare gradum superasque euadere ad auras,
> *hoc opus, hic labor est.*

On the other hand Ovid is not likely to mock Virgil in a hostile spirit (his admiration for him is stated several times and shown practically in the *Metamorphoses*). Rather this is the kind of parody which involves mocking one's own pretensions (Kenney in *Ovidiana*, p. 201).

**454. dederit :** in an erotic sense. As part of the same vocabulary note *negare* (345), *nolle* and *uelle* (274), *rogare* (277), *tangere* (92).

**457. littera Cydippen pomo perlata fefellit :** The young man Acontius inscribed on an apple 'I swear by Artemis to marry Acontius', and rolled it in front of Cydippe, who picked up the apple, read the words and was bound by the oath—remember that the ancients normally read aloud. This story formed perhaps the most celebrated episode in Callimachus' *Aetia* (frs. 67–75

Pfeiffer) and represents the whole of the poem at *Remedia* 382.
For a curious collection of inscriptions on apples, see A. R.
Littlewood, *Harvard Studies* 72 (1968), 167–8.

**459–62.** Cicero had recommended a broad training in the liberal
arts for a prospective orator (e.g. *Brutus* 322 ff., *Orator* 113 ff.).
Ovid agrees, but would put the resulting rhetorical skill to a
very different use (462)!

**459. disce bonas artes, moneo, Romana iuuentus :** His tone is
grandiloquent in the extreme (recalling *Georgics* ii. 35–6 'quare
agite o proprios generatim discite cultus, / agricolae'), aided by
the fact that Father Ennius had ended a hexameter with
'Romana iuuentus' at least three times (*Annals* 480, 489, 529
Warmington). Horace picks up the clausula, also in a mock-
heroic style, at *Sat.* ii. 2. 52.

**bonas artes :** the arts appropriate to a free-born man, called
alternatively *artes ingenuae, liberales*, or *honestae*. These would
include such studies as literature, mathematics, and music—
not, in the present context, rhetoric, but rather the general
education which will make a complete orator (compare Tacitus,
*Dialogus* 30. 4 'in libris Ciceronis deprehendere licet non geo-
metriae, non musicae, non grammaticae, non denique ullius
ingenuae artis scientiam ei defuisse').

**460. trepidos ut tueare reos :** Here and in the next line we see the
traditional eulogy of a public-spirited man of affairs. Compare
Horace on Pollio 'insigne maestis praesidium reis / et consulenti,
Pollio, curiae' (*Odes* ii. 1. 13–14, also *Odes* iv. 1. 14 on Paullus
Fabius Maximus) and Cornelius Severus on Cicero himself (fr.
13. 12–14 Morel) 'unica sollicitis quondam tutela salusque, /
egregium semper patriae caput, ille senatus / uindex, ille fori'.

**461. quam populus iudexque grauis lectusque senatus :** The three-
fold division denotes successively haranguing the people in a
*contio*, forensic oratory, and speaking before the Senate.

**iudexque grauis :** We should probably think of a single judge
sitting alone, as in perhaps a majority of private cases. Ovid
himself performed this function (*Tristia* ii. 95 'res quoque
priuatas statui sine crimine iudex'—see further Kenney, *Yale
Classical Studies* 21 (1969), 248–9).

**lectusque senatus :** *Lectio Senatus* was performed by the
Censor, who read over the names of members, striking out un-
worthy ones; cf. Livy ix. 29 'infamem atque inuidiosam senatus
lectionem'. Augustus writes 'senatum ter legi' (*Res Gestae* 8)—
this was very necessary after the Civil War period when num-
bers had become grossly inflated and many unworthy Senators
had gained admittance.

**462. dabit . . . manus :** a favourite Ovidian phrase. The gesture is
one of holding out the hands in submission.

**463–8.** *The style of your letter.* Ovid seems to be straying towards rhetorical theory when he warns against affectation (464) and unusual words (467). But even the art of letter-writing had its technical literature. In Demetrius, *On Style* (? late Hellenistic or early Roman period), paragraphs 223–35 (translated by Miss D. C. Innes in Russell and Winterbottom, *Ancient Literary Criticism* (1972), pp. 211–12) are devoted to the theory of letter-writing, and the precepts resemble those here quite closely. A letter should reveal the writer's character, and—though Demetrius has certain reservations—be like one side of a dialogue (cf. Ovid 468). The style must be plain (cf. 464) and the structure free; a letter should not imitate a speech in the law-courts (cf. 463), nor be too declamatory (cf. 465).

**463. in fronte :** 'ostentatiously'.

**464. uerba molesta :** 'laboured' or 'affected', cf. Suetonius, *Div. Aug.* 86 'opus est dare te operam ne moleste scribas et loquaris' and the use of 'molestiae' in Cicero, *Brutus* 315.

**466. saepe ualens odii littera causa fuit :** I would somewhat prefer to attach 'ualens' to 'littera' (cf. Seneca, *Contr.* iii. *Praef.* 2 'oratio eius erat ualens') although the decision is marginal (for 'causa ualens' compare e.g. *Met.* v. 174).

**467. credibilis sermo :** 'plausible', 'convincing', just as Greek rhetoric constantly stresses the need to be πιθανός.

consuetaque uerba : one of the commonest rhetorical precepts, to avoid archaic, abstruse, or invented words. Caesar urged 'ut tamquam scopulum sic fugias inauditum atque insolens uerbum' (*ap.* Gellius i. 10. 4, cf. e.g. Cicero, *de Oratore* iii. 39, C. O. Brink, *Horace on Poetry, The 'Ars Poetica'* (Cambridge, 1971) p. 133).

**469 ff.** Three possible reactions to your letter are envisaged, starting with the worst: (a) she sends the letter back unopened (469–78), (b) she reads it and makes no reply (479–82), (c) she replies, but in harsh tones, asking you to be good enough not to trouble her (483–6).

**470. propositumque tene :** i.e. continue to write. One is tempted here to find an echo of yet another famous piece of national poetry (cf. 453 n.), for Horace had extolled the 'tenacem propositi uirum' (*Odes* iii. 3. 1).

**471–6.** These examples of time's gradual effect are trite enough to need no illustration. But note the very similar passage in a similar context at Tibullus i. 4. 17–20 (K. F. Smith ad loc. collects parallels).

**472. lenta . . . frena :** 'pliant reins' (more often 'frena' = 'bit' or 'bridle', as at 20).

**475–6.** This not very striking couplet is quoted by Seneca (*Q.N.* iv b. 3) and misquoted among the Pompeian graffiti (*C.I.L.* IV. 1895 = *Carmina Latina Epigraphica* 1936. 1–2).

477. Penelope represents not a faithful wife, as she usually does, but merely a difficult proposition.

478. **capta uides sero Pergama, capta tamen** : The Greeks' ten-year siege of Troy became proverbial for effort rewarded (Theocritus 15. 61 ἐς Τροίαν πειρώμενοι ἦνθον Ἀχαιοί).

479. **legerit et nolit rescribere** : 'suppose she has read it and refuses to reply'. Martial (ii. 9) makes an elegant epigram from this predicament:

> scripsi; rescripsit nil Naeuia; non dabit ergo.
> at, puto, quod scripsi legerat: ergo dabit.

482. **ueniunt** : a general statement—'these things happen in their own good time' (Kenney).

483. **tristis** : 'harsh'.

485. **quod non rogat, optat, ut instes** : i.e. optat ut instes id quod non rogat, 'she wants you to press on with what she does not ask for' (cf. *Aeneid* viii. 433-4 'Marti currumque rotasque uolucris / instabant').

487 ff. *How to behave while you are conducting this tricky correspondence.* You have now declared yourself by letter, and must take every opportunity to be near your beloved. So the scene returns to the colonnades and theatres where Ovid first recommended that you should find a girl (67 ff.).

487. **siue illa toro resupina feretur** : She is carried comfortably reclining in a litter borne by slaves (see Mayor on Juvenal i. 64); this would have curtains that could be opened or shut at will (cf. Juvenal i. 124 'ostendens uacuam et clausam pro coniuge sellam').

488. **lecticam dominae dissimulanter adi** : For a less favourable view of such activities, contrast Martial v. 61. 3-4 on the false *procurator* 'nescio quid dominae teneram qui garrit in aurem / et sellam cubito dexteriore premit' and iii. 63. 7-8 on Cotilus 'inter femineas tota qui luce cathedras / desidet atque aliqua semper in aure sonat'.

490. **qua potes** : preferable to 'quam potes' (Kenney, *CQ* 1959, 249).

491. **uacuis** : 'at leisure'.

493-4. All these manoeuvres will conceal your purpose from the world at large.

495. **de mediis** : of the pillars in the colonnade which separate you from her.

498. **quod spectes, umeris adferet illa suis** : You must pay more attention to her pretty face than to the entertainment on stage. Ovid may glance at the proverb 'to carry on one's shoulders' meaning 'to bear responsibility for' (Otto, *Sprichwörter*, s.v. Umerus).

**499. respicias :** According to the emperor's prescription women sat segregated in the back rows of the theatre (see on 109 'respiciunt').

**500.** The hidden language of a sign or a gesture figures prominently in ancient love-poetry, above all in banquet scenes (thus 569 ff.).

**501–2.** A couplet containing more than meets the eye. Ovid surely refers to the mime (though Reynolds, *CQ* 1946, 79 n. 1 appears to doubt this), which he mentions at *Tristia* ii. 497 ff. as a more immoral type of literature than anything he had ever written himself. Mime regularly presented a triangular situation involving a woman, her idiotic husband, and her lover ('in quibus assidue cultus procedit adulter, / uerbaque dat stulto callida nupta uiro', *Tristia* ii. 499–500). And the point of the show lay in the clever stratagems with which the lover outwitted the husband (ibid. 505–6 'cumque fefellit amans aliqua nouitate maritum / plauditur et magno palma fauore datur'); see R. W. Reynolds, 'The Adultery Mime', *CQ* 40 (1946), 77–84. So when the young man here applauds the actor playing the female part (501) and shows his support for the lover in the plot (502), the girl is meant to get the message. In fact these lines seem to portray the woman as married, in accord with a tradition of Latin love-elegy rather than with Ovid's own profession at 31–4 (see further Introduction pp. xv–xvii).

More information on the Mime can be found in W. Beare, *The Roman Stage*[3], particularly pp. 149–58, and Owen's note on *Tristia* ii. 497 ff.

**501. aliquam mimo saltante puellam :** Although women had played female parts probably from the start of mime in Italy (Beare, op. cit., p. 152), it was no less common for these to be taken by men, as here. Beare (ibid.) quotes the epitaph of a *mimus* who claimed that he could play either sex equally well. The Christian writers attack this feature in addition to the overall licentiousness of the genre (Arnobius, *adv. Nat.* vii. 33 'iam uero si uiderint in femineas mollitudines eneruantes se uiros . . . manus ad caelum tollunt').

**502. faueas :** Individual actors had their fans, and the enthusiasm shown in the theatre might be tremendous (e.g. Cicero, *pro Rosc. Com.* 29 'quod studium et quem fauorem secum in scaenam attulit Panurgus').

**504. arbitrio dominae tempora perde tuae :** I suspect that it was the frivolity of the *Ars* (shown in lines like this) which was intended to upset traditional Roman sentiment. Romans had strong ideas about the use of time, as Ovid himself acknowledges at *Tristia* ii. 483–4 'quique alii lusus . . . / perdere, rem caram, tempora nostra solent', cf. Horace, *Odes* i. 1. 20 'nec partem solido demere de die'.

**505 ff.** At this point Ovid is in danger of recommending too dandi-
fied a mode of behaviour, and so he hastens to redress the
balance by insisting on a more masculine ideal. The way of life
against which he warns is well exemplified by Martial's 'bellus
homo' Cotilus (iii. 63. 3–12):

> bellus homo est, flexos qui digerit ordine crines,
>     balsama qui semper, cinnama semper olet;
> cantica qui Nili, qui Gaditana susurrat,
>     qui mouet in uarios bracchia uolsa modos;
> inter femineas tota qui luce cathedras
>     desidet atque aliqua semper in aure sonat,
> qui legit hinc illinc missas scribitque tabellas;
>     pallia uicini qui refugit cubiti;
> qui scit quam quis amet, qui per conuiuia currit,
>     Hirpini ueteres qui bene nouit auos.

**505. sed tibi nec ferro placeat torquere capillos :** Men did curl their
hair at Rome, but this was considered foppish (e.g. Cicero, *pro
Sestio* 18).

**ferro :** with the curling-iron or *calamistrum*.

**torquere :** 'twist', but also with the implication of 'torturing'
the hair into unnatural curls.

**506.** Ovid's sensibility is supported by Seneca on paying too much
and too little attention to rhetorical style—'ille et crura, hic ne
alas quidem uellit' (*Epist.* 114. 14).

**507–8.** Such things may be left to the eunuch priests of the Magna
Mater. This was the first Eastern cult to reach Rome, at the end
of the third century B.C. (see Fordyce's introduction to Catullus
63). Its votaries must have been a familiar sight in procession
through the streets of Rome and other Italian cities (cf. Lucre-
tius ii. 610 ff.) but they were undoubtedly viewed with some
contempt (see Pease on *Aeneid* iv. 215). In Ovid's time no
Roman citizen would be a priest of Cybele.

**507. Cybeleia mater :** the Phrygian Great Mother, Cybele (or
Cybebe); her priests were known as *galli*.

**508. exululata :** Ecstatic cries show the frenzied nature of her rites
(cf. Catullus 63. 24 'ubi sacra sancta acutis ululatibus agitant',
Maecenas fr. 6 Morel 'latus horreat flagello, comitum chorus
ululet'). 'Ululare' is an onomatopoeic word like ὀλολυγμός in
Greek.

**509–12.** Ovid speaks with the same voice as Cicero (*de Officiis* i.
130 'a forma remoueatur omnis uiro non dignus ornatus') and,
later, Quintilian on the appropriate dress for an orator—'sit . . .
splendidus et uirilis: nam et toga et calceus et capillus tam nimia
cura quam neglegentia sunt reprehendenda' (*Inst. Or.* xi. 3.
137). Apparently Philaenis περὶ ἀφροδισίων also recommended that

a lover should neglect his appearance, but for a different pur-
pose—to conceal his intentions from their object (*P. Oxy.* 39
(1972), no. 2891).

**509. Minoida** : Ariadne.

**510. abstulit** : 'swept off her feet' (and in a secondary sense
'carried away from her home'), cf. Virgil, *Ecl.* 8. 41 'ut uidi, ut
perii, ut me malus abstulit error!'

**511.** In the *Heroides* (4. 75 ff.) Phaedra compliments Hippolytus
on not taking too much trouble over his appearance: 'sint
procul a nobis iuuenes ut femina compti! / fine coli modico
forma uirilis amat. / te tuus iste rigor positique sine arte capilli /
et leuis egregio puluis in ore decet.'

**512. Adonis** : the hunter, beloved of Venus.

**513–24.** A most interesting passage—how the Society man was
dressed and groomed in 2 B.C. Other Roman writings indicate
that these lines owe little to elegiac convention; they represent
the typical Roman opinion of the time as to decent personal
appearance. In one respect, as we shall see (729 n.), the conven-
tion of love-poetry was just the opposite. The ancients were on
the whole more sensitive to standards of appearance and out-
ward behaviour than we are; deviations from the norm, besides
offering an easy target for ridicule, might suggest moral or even
political turpitude.

Even in so truly Roman a context Ovid follows the didactic
tradition: to state physical and sartorial requirements for the
job was by no means alien to didactic verse. Compare first
Hesiod, *Works and Days* 536 ff., and much later Oppian, *Cyn.* i.
81 ff. (culminating in 108 ὧδε μὲν εὖ στέλλοιντο θοὸν δέμας ἀγρευτῆρες
'and thus should hunters well equip their nimble bodies') and
*Hal.* iii. 29 ff., where the poet recommends that a fisherman be
strong, swift of foot, neither too fat nor too thin (πρῶτα μὲν ἀσπαλιῆι
δέμας καὶ γυῖα παρείη / ἀμφότερον καὶ κραιπνὰ καὶ ἄλκιμα, μήτε τι λίην / πίονα
μήτε τι σαρκὶ λελειμμένα).

**513. munditie placeant** : The quality of *munditia* or *mundities* is
not easily caught in English. It applies more often to women
(e.g. Horace, *Odes* i. 5. 5) than to men, and may be far from
complimentary of the latter, e.g. Seneca, *Contr.* i, *praef.* 8
'mollitia corporis certare cum feminis et immundissimis se
expolire munditiis nostrorum adulescentium specimen est.'
Cicero (*de Officiis* i. 130) strikes the right note of caution: 'adhi-
benda praeterea munditia est non odiosa neque exquisita nimis,
tantum quae fugiat agrestem et inhumanam neglegentiam.'
Here too the emphasis must be on *restrained* elegance (similarly in
Nepos, *Atticus* 13. 5 'munditiam, non adfluentiam adfectabat').

A small problem of text and interpretation arises. With the
punctuation printed, *corpora* is subject of *placeant* as well as of

*fuscentur*; this seems preferable to putting a colon after *placeant* and making its subject 'uiri' understood from 'uiros' in 509. There remains a question whether Ovid is likely to have used the fifth-declension *mundities* here (older editors printed *munditiae* as nominative plural). In general the fifth-declension forms have a slightly old-fashioned tone—Lucretius was particularly fond of them (see Bailey's edition, vol. I, pp. 74 and 79–80). Housman remarked that Ovid only uses the first-declension form 'duritia' in the *Heroides*, and 'duritiem' at *Met.* i. 401 is probably meant to have an archaic ring (as Lee suggests). But 'mollities' seems secure at *Am.* iii. 8. 18, and so we need not doubt the likelihood of 'mundities' here.

**fuscentur corpora Campo** : You should have a healthy suntan from exercising in the Campus Martius. As Cicero puts it (*de Off.* i. 130) 'formae autem dignitas coloris bonitate tuenda est, color exercitationibus corporis'. These exercises would include gymnastics, horsemanship, the handling of weapons, swimming in the Tiber and various ball-games; cf. iii. 383–6 'sunt illis (sc. the men) celeresque pilae iaculumque trochique / armaque et in gyros ire coactus equus; / nec uos Campus habet nec uos gelidissima Virgo / nec Tuscus placida deuehit amnis aqua' and Horace, *Odes* i. 8 with the commentary of Nisbet and Hubbard.

**Campo** : Platner and Ashby (*Topographical Dictionary*, s.v. Campus Martius) note that in Augustus' time the Campus was divided into two parts—the area between the cippus and the Circus Flaminius, which had already begun to be built over, and the remaining open meadow to the north, the Campus proper.

**514–18.** In *Satires* i. 3. 31–2 Horace lists three ways of making yourself ridiculous, all of which recur here—if your hair is inexpertly cut, if your toga falls off the shoulder, or if your shoes are too big, 'rusticius tonso toga defluit, et male laxus / in pede calceus haeret' (cf. *Epist.* i. 1. 94–6, Juvenal 3. 149 'si toga sordidula est').

**514. sit bene conueniens et sine labe toga** : Of course the 'gens togata' (*Aen.* i. 282) took a particular pride in their national dress—Hortensius is even said to have prosecuted a colleague who bumped into him and disarranged its folds (Macrobius iii. 13. 5)! Quintilian gives detailed instructions for the orator's toga (xi. 3. 137 ff.). To make it fit exactly was by no means easy, as he admits (ibid. 139 'ipsam togam rutundam esse et apte caesam uelim, aliter enim multis modis fiet enormis') and Tertullian, arguing for the Christian *pallium*, sarcastically asks wearers of the toga whether they think they are dressed or laden (*de Pallio* 5. 1). In modern times Lillian M. Wilson devoted a whole book to the Roman Toga (Baltimore, 1924).

**515.** †lingua ne rigeat† ; careant rubigine dentes : The first half of this line presents a very difficult problem. One naturally assumes that both statements refer to oral hygiene, and Kenney, following the idea of A. G. Lee and W. M. Edwards, hesitantly put forward 'gingiuae niteant', 'let your gums sparkle' (other suggestions along the same lines are less attractive). We would then have a parallel for iii. 197 'ne fuscet inertia dentes', and *robigo* can denote a scabrous film on teeth (*Met*. ii. 776).

But it is strange that 514 should describe the toga and 516 the sandals with an intervening line on oral hygiene; not counting 515 Ovid seems to review general features and clothing before more intimate details. Palmer cleverly emended 'lingua' to 'lingula', i.e. the tongue of a shoe. He further suggested 'ruget' for 'rigeat', comparing iii. 444 'breuis in rugas lingula pressa suas'. But, as Goold rightly points out (*Harvard Studies* 69 (1965), 65–6), that line indicates that it *was* smart to have the tongue of your shoe creased. So he preferred 'lingula ne rigeat', 'do not let the tongue of your shoe be stiff', with a minimal change of the manuscripts. It will then be necessary to refer 'dentes' to the 'teeth' of a shoe-buckle. While we have no supporting evidence for this (Festus p. 103, 21–3 Lindsay, quoted by Goold, helps not at all on *dens*), it is far from unreasonable—the word is used elsewhere of e.g. a comb and a bit.

**516.** nec uagus in laxa pes tibi pelle natet : on having too big shoes cf. Horace, *Sat*. i. 3. 31–2 (quoted on 514–18). Theophrastus (*Characters* 4) attributes this to the boorish man (ἄγροικος).

natet : 'swim', the same figure as at Aristophanes, *Knights* 321 ἔνεον ἐν ταῖς ἐμβάσιν.

**517.** Compare Horace, *Sat*. i. 3. 31 (above) and *Epist*. i. 1. 94–5 'si curatus inaequali tonsore capillos / occurri, rides.'

**518.** sit coma, sit trita barba resecta manu : Young men in Ovid's day would sport a small, neat beard; the full, thick one associated with the old Republic came back in the time of Hadrian. Compare Cicero, *pro Caelio* 33 'aliquis mihi ab inferis excitandus est ex barbatis illis, non hac barbula qua ista delectatur sed illa horrida quam in statuis antiquis atque imaginibus uidemus' and Austin ad loc. For the social and moral significance of hair style and length, see Christopher Ehrhardt, 'Hair in Ancient Greece', in *Classical News and Views* 15. 1 (January 1971), 13–19; he mentions two further articles in the same periodical, G. Bagnani 'Misopogon, the Beard Hater' (Oct. 1968, 73–9) and B. Baldwin, 'Some Roman Hairs Apparent' (Jan. 1969, 26–7).

trita : 'practised' (thus 'tritiores manus', Vitruvius ii. 1. 6, and 'tritae aures', Cicero, *ad Fam*. ix. 16. 4). This is Housman's correction (*CR* 4 (1890), 341–2), closer to the manuscripts than 'scita' (Heinsius).

**519.** The Roman barber also gave a careful manicure; at Horace, *Epist.* i. 7. 50–1 it is cause for comment that Vulteius Mena does this for himself, 'uacua tonsoris in umbra / cultello proprios purgantem leniter ungues'. Overlong finger-nails are attributed by Theophrastus to the δυσχερής, the man who offends others (*Characters* 19), cf. Horace, *Ars Poetica* 297 'bona pars non unguis ponere curat.'

**522. uirque paterque gregis** : i.e. a he-goat—an intentionally absurd use of the elaborate periphrasis, not unlike Horace, *Odes* i. 17. 7 'olentis uxores mariti' (see Nisbet and Hubbard ad loc.).

**524. male uir** : together, 'of doubtful masculinity'.

**525–6.** A sharp break pointed by 'ecce' (525). We are told that Bacchus can help lovers in the passion which he too has felt; it emerges at 565 ff. that the god represents wine by metonymy, and the scene has shifted to a party (briefly anticipated at 229 ff.). But, however tenuous the connexion, it serves to introduce a most attractive digression on the abandonment of Ariadne and her rescue by Bacchus.

**525. suum uatem** : Dionysus shared with Apollo the patronage of poetry, cf. [Tibullus] iii. 4. 43–4 'casto nam rite poetae / Phoebusque et Bacchus Pieridesque fauent.' There was also the idea, often directed against Callimachus and his admirers, that to be any good a poet must drink heavily—the work of 'aquae potores' (ὑδροπόται) would not survive (Horace, *Epist.* i. 19. 1 ff.).

**526. et flammae, qua calet ipse, fauet** : An appeal to the god's own experience in love had become commonplace (see Gow on Theocritus 8. 59 ff.). Meleager gave the motif an unusual twist when he brought in not the flame of love but the fiery thunderbolt which induced Bacchus' birth ἐν πυρὶ γεννηθεὶς στέργεις φλόγα τὰν ἐν Ἔρωτι (*Anth. Pal.* xii. 119 (= Meleager 20 Gow–Page). 3).

**527–64.** This passage (not requiring very detailed comment) can hardly be beaten for sheer gusto and high spirits. The abandonment of Ariadne by Theseus ranked among the most famous poetic situations; perhaps about A.D. 50 a minor practitioner ([Virgil], *Aetna* 21–2) asks 'quis non periurae doluit mendacia puppis / desertam uacuo Minoida litore questus?' Catullus 64, The Marriage of Peleus and Thetis, provides our best-known handling of the story, where Ariadne forms the inset digression; on the ground of similarities between Catullus and the late Greek poet Nonnus Fordyce (on Cat. 64. 139 and 160) suggests that the laments of Ariadne may already have been a set piece in Hellenistic poetry. See T. B. L. Webster, *Greece & Rome* 13 (1966), 22–31 for an illustrated account of the myth from Homer to Catullus.

The important point to recognize is that a treatment of the

Ariadne legend would almost invariably contain a long mono-
logue by the abandoned girl—and this might become very
stereotyped. So many mythical heroines had been deserted by
their lovers that the reproaches of a Phyllis, an Ariadne, a
Medea, or even a Dido inevitably seemed much of a muchness.
Ovid now takes up quite a different position. He is not con-
cerned to give Ariadne's words at length, nor even to move our
sympathy for her plight—quite the reverse. Indeed she protests
and indeed she weeps (533), but this only makes her look prettier.
We are given just a snatch of her lament (536–7); no sooner has
she repeated 'what will become of me?' than the music of the
Bacchants is heard off-stage (537)—Ariadne did not have to
wait long before her question was answered. One might quote
the words which Ovid gives her at *Fasti* iii. 463–4 '"quid
flebam rustica?" dixit / "utiliter nobis perfidus ille fuit."' Of
course the context here demands that the poet should concen-
trate on Ariadne's rescue by Bacchus rather than her complaint,
but this gives an unusual turn and an extra spice to the
episode.

**527. Cnosis :** 'the girl from Cnossos', as 556 'Cnosias'.

**528. Dia :** the island, later identified with Naxos (Callimachus fr.
601) where Artemis kills Ariadne in Homer (*Odyssey* xi. 325).
Homer's version appears to be quite different: Ariadne has been
married to Dionysus, but leaves him for the mortal Theseus.

**529.** 'Just as she was straight from her sleep, clothed in an un-
girdled tunic' (cf. Catullus 64. 56–7 'utpote fallaci quae tum
primum excita somno / desertam in sola miseram se cernat
harena'). For the picture of her disarray compare ibid. 63–5 'non
flauo retinens subtilem uertice mitram, / non contecta leui uela-
tum pectus amictu, / non tereti strophio lactentis uincta papillas'.
    **e somno :** as e.g. Catullus 63. 36 'nimio e labore'.

**530. croceas . . . comas :** fair-haired like a good epic heroine (cf.
Hesiod, *Theogony* 947 ξανθὴν Ἀριάδνην).

**531. Thesea crudelem :** She cries 'crudelis Theseu', or, as in
Catullus, 'perfide' (64. 132–3, ibid. 137–8 'tibi nulla fuit cle-
mentia praesto, / immite ut nostri uellet miserescere pectus?').
Compare *Fasti* iii. 473 'dicebam, memini, "periure et perfide
Theseu"' and 536 below.

**533. sed utrumque decebat :** a common motif, as at 126 of the
Sabine women.

**536. quid mihi fiet? :** Catullus (64. 177 ff.) makes her ask rhetori-
cally 'nam quo me referam? quali spe perdita nitor? etc.', and
she concludes (186–7) 'nulla fugae ratio, nulla spes: omnia
muta, / omnia sunt deserta, ostentant omnia letum.' In the
*Heroides* (10. 83 ff.) she speculates about other inhabitants of
the island: 'iam iam uenturos aut hac aut suspicor illac / qui

lanient auido uiscera dente lupos; / forsitan et fuluos tellus alat
ista leones; / quis scit an et saeuam tigrida Dia ferat?'

**537.** At this point we begin to hear the approach of the god's
retinue (compare Catullus 64. 251 ff. 'at parte ex alia florens
uolitabat Iacchus / cum thiaso Satyrorum et Nysigenis Silenis, /
te quaerens, Ariadna, tuoque incensus amore etc.'). Ovid re-
serves the god himself for an impressive entrance at the end
(549).

**538. adtonita tympana pulsa manu :** Alliteration is frequent in
such ecstatic descriptions; the pattern here with *t* and *p* is
paralleled at Lucretius ii. 618 'tympana tenta tonant palmis' of
the followers of Cybele. Our poet excels in dropping just momen-
tarily into a given style.

**539. excidit :** 'She fainted.'

**541. Mimallonides :** a Macedonian term for the Bacchants, per-
haps popularized by Callimachus (fr. 503—note also Euphorion
*P. Oxy.* 2219 fr. 3. 15). It is obviously most exquisite; compare
one of the lines mocked by Persius (1. 99) 'torua Mimalloneis
inplerunt cornua bombis.'

   **sparsis in terga capillis :** Dishevelled locks due to wild tossing
of the head backwards regularly characterize these ladies (see
Dodds on Euripides, *Bacchae* 862–5).

**543–8.** E. de St. Denis in *Ovidiana* (opposite p. 198) shows a
mosaic from Pompeii of Silenus carrying a staff and riding
inebriated upon a donkey with two Satyrs in close attendance.
The animal seems to have collapsed beneath the old man's
weight, and the two Satyrs are trying to set it on its feet, grasping
it the one by its tail, the other by its ears. De St. Denis wonders
whether the mosaic could be inspired by Ovid—this is possible,
but of course both versions could derive from Hellenistic poetry
or art.

**544. arte :** ironical—in fact he can barely stay on by grasping the
mane.

**545.** Understand 'dum' also with 'Bacchae fugiuntque petuntque'
(presumably the Bacchae provoke Silenus by running towards
him and then away); 547 forms the main clause of the sentence.

**546. quadrupedem :** contemptuously 'the creature', as e.g. Apu-
leius, *Met.* vii. 27 'quadrupes nequissime'.

**549.** Enter the god, altogether more purposeful and skilful than
Silenus.

   **quem summum texerat uuis :** In the Ptolomaic pageant de-
scribed by Athenaeus (v. 198d) the carriage of Dionysus bore
a canopy decorated with ivy, vine, and other fruits.

**550. tigribus adiunctis :** The tigers proclaim him an Eastern
conqueror (see on 189–90); elsewhere Bacchus' chariot is drawn
by lynxes (e.g. Propertius iii. 17. 8). In fact the Greeks only met

the tiger in the Hellenistic age. Seleucus I presented a specimen to the Athenians (see Athenaeus xiii. 590a for allusions to it in the comic poets Philemon and Alexis); another early and striking mention of the tiger occurs in Euphorion, where, if the restoration is correct, Justice 'moves like a tiger' in pursuit of wrongdoers (Page, Loeb *Greek Literary Papyri* (Poetry), p. 496, 21).

**551. et color et Theseus et uox abiere puellae :** a particularly fine example of Ovidian syllepsis, as Professor Kenney would have us call it (see his note on Lucretius iii. 614). Observe too the irony in 'Theseus left her'—he had already done so in a different sense.

**552. terque . . . terque :** a conventional pattern (see Pease on *Aeneid* iv. 690).

**553. steriles . . . aristas :** The epithet is puzzling—the only attempt to explain it which I have seen is that of Heinsius, 'sole adustas et proinde steriles', comparing *Heroides* 5. 111–12 'et minus est in te quam summa pondus arista, / quae leuis assiduis solibus usta riget' (possibly add Claudian, *in Eutropium* i. 116 'ieiunae . . . aristae'); he also considered reading 'auenae' (-as), for which 'sterilis' is a common epithet. Goold (*Harvard Studies* 69 (1965), 66) would emend to 'graciles', quoting in support *Amores* i. 7. 55 and *Heroides* 14. 39. If change is thought necessary I prefer 'fragiles' as a dry and brittle word, contrasting with the moist and muddy picture in 554 (for such an artistic contrast in double similes see my note on *Met.* viii. 835–9). With Goold (ibid.) I would print 'aristae' rather than 'aristas' at the end of the line.

**555.** For 'cura' of the beloved one cf. 512 and Virgil, *Ecl.* 10. 22.

**557. munus habe caelum :** as he says to her in Nonnus (xlvii. 447) οὐρανὸν οἶκον ἔχεις. See *Oxf. Lat. Dict.* s.v. 5a for 'munus' as a gift on special occasions (e.g. a wedding).

**557–8.** The 'catasterism' of Ariadne's crown is a well-known legend (e.g. *Met.* viii. 177–82), but Ovid seems to do an unusual thing here in combining it with a much rarer account whereby Ariadne herself is raised to the skies ('caelo spectabere sidus', cf. *Fasti* iii. 509 ff. where she becomes the Italian goddess Libera, Propertius iii. 17. 8). Even so, *reget* in 558 is preferable to *reges* (which would make an uncomfortably close identification of Ariadne with her crown). The former was conjectured by Merkel and is in fact the reading of Y, while R and O have 'rege'; almost certainly the common ancestor of the α' group had 'reget' (Kenney, *CR* 1966, 268).

**560. (inposito cessit harena pede) :** because the god is larger and heavier than a mortal, cf. *Fasti* iii. 330 'terraque subsedit pondere pressa Iouis.'

**562. in facili est omnia posse deo** : an amusing aside, which indi-
cates that readers may not find winning their girl quite so
simple! Homer has a phrase ῥεῖα μάλ' ὥς τε θεός ('very easily,
like a god', e.g. *Iliad* iii. 381).

**563.** Some raise the marriage-cry 'Hymenaee' (for a discussion of
which see Fordyce's introduction to Catullus 61, Costa on
Seneca, *Medea* 56-115 and 67-70) and others the Bacchic shout
'Euhion, euhoe' (cf. Catullus 64. 255 'euhoe bacchantes, euhoe
capita inflectentes').

**565 ff.** The connection with what has gone before is a little weak,
and Ovid tries to patch it by some verbal juggling. He picks up
'toro' (564) with 'tori' (566). 'Positi . . . Bacchi' (565), 'wine set
before you', recalls the god reclining with Ariadne—similarly
'in socii femina parte tori' (566). This rather awkward transition
takes us to a banquet where your young lady is sharing a couch
with you. The advice which follows is predictable; such motifs
as tracing messages in wine on the table are familiar e.g. from
Tibullus, but the main source for this passage is Ovid's own
poem, *Amores* i. 4. There he proposes to attend a banquet with
his girl, and instructs her how to behave, particularly how to
outwit her 'uir'. Ovid also mentions the 'uir' at 579 ff. below,
but in the present case his advice to the lover is quite differ-
ent. For party games from the female point of view compare iii.
749 ff.

That such a scene did have some plausibility in contemporary
Rome is suggested by Horace, *Odes* iii. 6. 25 ff., a serious poem
which would lose in force if the illustration were purely con-
ventional and derived from Greek sympotic poetry. Horace tells
how young women blatantly look for lovers at the drinking-
parties of their complaisant husbands:

> mox iuniores quaerit adulteros
> inter mariti uina, neque eligit
>     cui donet impermissa raptim
>     oscula luminibus remotis,
>
> sed iussa coram non sine conscio
> surgit marito, seu uocat institor
>     seu nauis Hispanae magister,
>     dedecorum pretiosus emptor.

**565. ergo** : drawing the moral from previous lines in didactic
fashion (cf. 343).

**567. Nycteliumque patrem** : the title of Bacchus whose cere-
monies take place at night (from νύξ and perhaps τελεῖν, making
a link with 'nocturnaque sacra'), cf. *Met.* iv. 15, [Virgil], *Culex*
111, Nonnus, *Dionysiaca* xxii. 6.

**nocturnaque sacra :** at Euripides, *Bacchae* 485–6 Dionysus, asked whether he performs his rites by day or night, replies νύκτωρ τὰ πολλά.

**569–70.** *Your conversation should be deliberately ambiguous,* as illustrated in line 601.

**571–2.** Tracing love messages in wine on the table is one of the motifs which Ovid claims at *Tristia* ii. 454 (see Owen ad loc.) can equally be found in Tibullus—he refers to Tib. i. 6. 19–20. Compare *Amores* i. 4. 20 'uerba notata mero', *Heroides* 17. 89–90 'orbe quoque in mensae legi sub nomine nostro / quod deducta mero littera fecit "amo".'

**575–6. fac primus rapias illius tacta labellis / pocula, quaque bibet parte puella, bibas :** When the ancients drank a toast, the cup was passed round those involved, cf. Plautus, *Asinaria* 771–2 'tecum una postea aeque pocla potitet, / aps ted accipiat, tibi propinet', Juvenal 5. 127–9 'quando propinat / Virro tibi sumitue tuis contacta labellis / pocula ?', *Amores* i. 4. 31–2. In Greek the epigram of Agathias is justly famous: εἰμὶ μὲν οὐ φιλόοινος ὅταν δ' ἐθέλῃς με μεθύσσαι, / πρῶτα σὺ γευομένη πρόσφερε, καὶ δέχομαι. / εἰ γὰρ ἐπιψαύσεις τοῖς χείλεσιν, οὐκέτι νήφειν / εὐμαρές, οὐδὲ φυγεῖν τὸν γλυκὺν οἰνοχόον (*Anth. Pal.* v. 261. 1–4 'I am not fond of wine, but if you wish to make me drunk, first do you taste and bring me the cup, and then I will accept it. For if you touch it with your lips it is no longer easy to stay sober or to refuse the delightful wine-bearer').

**579 ff.** The *uir* comes in from *Amores* i. 4. Since Ovid professedly writes for *meretrices* (cf. 31–4, 435) he ought strictly to have removed from this work the 'husband' who is rival to the hero; that he did not do so is one more indication of the unreality of the genre. Probably Ovid was unwilling to abandon some poetically promising situations, at whatever risk of being misunderstood or misrepresented. See further Introduction pp. xvi–xvii.

Two very witty poems in the *Amores* feature the *uir*. In ii. 19 Ovid complains unexpectedly that the *uir* is not looking after his wife with sufficient care—'your lack of opposition is ruining my game'; the finale is a master-paradox: 'if you want me to be your rival (as apparently you do) then tell me not to be.' By contrast *Amores* iii. 4 is addressed to an old-fashioned husband who has set a guard on his wife. Ovid delivers a solemn moral lecture along the line 'you may guard her body but her mind is unfaithful; a woman who is chaste because she has to be is not chaste at all.' He concludes 'why not accept all the friends whom your wife will bring you ? You will always be invited to parties by the young, and will see many presents at home that you have not had to pay for yourself.' In the same spirit here Ovid recommends that you should conciliate the *uir*.

**580. uobis :** to the pair of you.

**581. huic, si sorte bibes, sortem concede priorem :** What exactly is at stake here? If they are throwing to decide the order of drinking, Ovid may recommend either letting the *uir* have first throw, or allowing him to drink first in any event. It was also customary to throw for the office of symposiarch or governor of the feast (cf. Horace, *Odes* i. 4. 18 'nec regna uini sortiere talis' with Nisbet and Hubbard ad loc.), but I do not see how that practice could be relevant here.

**582. huic detur capiti missa corona tuo :** 'Give him the garland which has dropped from your head.' 'Missa' rather suggests that the garland has fallen accidentally (contrast ii. 528 'et capiti demptas in fore pone rosas'); in sympotic poetry the garland will often slip from the drinker's head as he becomes more inebriated (see J. Hangard, *Mnemosyne* 1971, 398–400), and here you are urged to place it on the husband's head as a token of good will.

   **corona :** The customary banqueter's garland plays a regular part in the serenade or *paraclausithyron*, when the lover finds his girl's front door barred to him, and after singing a mournful song departs, leaving the garland on a door-post (cf. ii. 528, quoted above, *Amores* i. 6. 67–8, Asclepiades, *Anth. Pal.* v. 145, Lucretius iv. 1178).

**584. nec dubites illi uerba secunda loqui :** probably a dramatic metaphor, cf. Horace, *Sat.* i. 9. 45–6 'haberes / magnum adiutorem, posset qui ferre secundas (sc. partes).' Ovid almost recommends that you should become a *scurra*, a kind of person who attached himself to another and flattered him by agreeing with all his opinions and applauding his dinner-table witticisms. Of course this would normally be thought a degrading part to play —hence 'nec dubites'.

**585–8.** These lines present a puzzling and intractable problem. The words 'crimen habet' (586) form an almost insuperable objection to accepting them here; in the middle of advising the lover to deceive the *uir*, Ovid can hardly draw attention to the moral blameworthiness of this act. On the other hand I would not wish to delete the lines as spurious—the double-edged use of legal and business terms in 587–8 is quite in our poet's manner (see on 83–6). Kenney suggested that the passage might be placed after 742, and in my opinion he stands a fair chance of being right. There 'crimen habet' would be appropriate enough; the lover has won his girl and is warned against the danger of losing her to a friend.

**585. tuta :** In any case 'trita' (Heinsius) is a plausible emendation here and in the next line (cf. 518). If we place these four lines after 742 (see above), 'trita' becomes essential in view of 'tutum' in 741.

**587. inde procurator nimium quoque multa procurat :** 'That is how the manager comes to manage too much.' A procurator, as defined by Ulpian (*Dig.* iii. 3. 1), 'aliena negotia mandatu [cf. 588] domini administrat'; cf. Cicero, *pro Caecina* 57 'procurator dicitur omnium rerum eius qui in Italia non sit absitue rei publicae causa quasi quidam paene dominus, hoc est alieni iuris uicarius.' He might be a friend and equal, as here, or perhaps more commonly someone of lower status, e.g. a freedman.

Reminiscent of this passage is Martial's epigram v. 61. After inquiring who is the doubtful young man always in attendance upon Marianus' wife, the poet learns that he is a *procurator* ('"uxoris res agit" inquis / "iste meae"') but counters with 'res uxoris agit? res ullas crispulus iste? / res non uxoris, res agit iste tuas' ('he is not doing your wife's business, but yours').

**prŏcurator :** the first syllable short as at *Fasti* iii. 343, Tibullus i. 5. 13 (long in Horace, *Epist.* i. 5. 21, Martial v. 61. 9). On similar uncertainties in Lucretius (e g. prŏpagare) see Bailey's edition, vol. I, p. 130.

**588. et sibi mandatis plura uidenda putat :** 'and sees fit to go beyond his commission'. Undoubtedly there is a double meaning in 'uidere', both to 'see to' or 'arrange' the business (e.g. Cicero, *ad Att.* v. 1. 3 'antecesserat Statius ut prandium nobis uideret') and to 'see' more of the lady than he should. Compare the playing with words in 83–6.

**mandatis :** a commission given by one person to another on a basis of trust.

**589–602.** *How much you should drink, and how you should and should not behave after wine.*

**589. certa tibi a nobis dabitur mensura bibendi :** in the pompous tone of some medical writer laying down the exact amount for a prescription.

**590. officium praestent mensque pedesque suum :** Compare Terence, *Eunuchus* 729 (on the effects of over-indulgence) 'postquam surrexi neque pes neque mens satis suom officium facit.'

**592. et nimium faciles ad fera bella manus :** Lenz (see the note in his Berlin 1969 edition) prefers the variant 'uerba' for 'bella', which was apparently in the copy used by Bishop Theodulf (cf. 36 n.); *ad* would then mean 'in response to' (as e.g. at *Fasti* iii. 536 'et iactant faciles ad sua uerba manus'), and *faciles* 'easily aroused'(cf. Lucan i. 173 'inde irae faciles'). In fact Heinsius gave a certain credence to 'uerba', which is not impossible but seems strained in comparison with 'bella'.

**593. Eurytion :** one of the Centaurs killed when, owing to excessive wine, the marriage-feast of Pirithous degenerated into a brawl; compare *Odyssey* xxi. 295–6 οἶνος καὶ Κένταυρον ἀγακλυτὸν Εὐρυτίωνα /

ἄασ' ἐνὶ μεγάρῳ μεγαθύμου Πειριθόοιο (the words οἶνος καὶ Κένταυρον became a proverb).

**595 ff.** Examples of amiable though slightly extravagant behaviour which will get by on such an occasion.

**595. si uox est, canta ; si mollia bracchia, salta :** The Bore who tried to commend himself to Horace boasted his accomplishments with 'quis membra mouere (sc. possit) / mollius? inuideat quod et Hermogenes ego canto' (*Sat.* i. 9. 24–5). In ancient dancing gesticulations with the arms were very important, so that χειρονομεῖν ('to move the hands') came to mean 'to dance'. But, although vigorous dancing was not unknown in early Rome (see on 112), it had once been a grievous insult to call a man a 'saltator'—'neque temere consulem populi Romani saltatorem uocare' (Cicero, *pro Murena* 13, cf. R. G. M. Nisbet on *in Pisonem* 18). To an extreme conservative singing might be little better: 'praeterea cantat' said the elder Cato of an adversary (Macrobius iii. 14, who also discusses dancing).

**598. titubet :** literally 'stagger', applied by a humorous turn to the tongue.

  **blaeso :** 'stammering'. The word is said properly to denote an inability to pronounce the sibilants *s* and *z*, which of course would apply well to drunkenness, real or feigned.

**599–600.** Very nicely illustrated in 601 (a line also containing the pointed ambiguity recommended at 569–70).

**601, bene dic dominae :** Say 'A health to the lady' (cf. Plautus, *Persa* 772[a] 'bene mihi, bene uobis, bene meae amicae'—one might also employ the accusative as in Tibullus ii. 1. 31 'bene Messalam'). Nobody could object to this: 'domina' was a polite and respectful term for a woman (whence *donna, dame*), but at the same time it regularly denotes the beloved mistress in Augustan love-poetry, so there is something of a *double entendre*.

  **bene, cum quo dormiat illa :** definitely in bad taste (*proteruius aequo*, 599), but that will be ascribed to your condition. Although the company would apply your words to the *uir*, you really mean yourself (cf. 602), and the girl gets the message.

**603 ff.** *When the party breaks up* (parallel to *Amores* i. 4. 55 ff.). This is your big chance, although Ovid declines to tell you what to say—the words will come of themselves (610).

**603. mensa . . . remota :** According to Roman custom separate tables would be brought on and taken away with each course, whence e.g. *mensae secundae* = the second course.

**606.** Compare Claudian, *in Eutropium* i. 85–6 'non blandior ullus euntis / ancillae tetigisse latus'.

**607–8. fuge rustice longe / hinc Pudor :** Cicero had described the shyness which prevented him from broaching a subject face to

face as 'pudor quidam paene subrusticus' (ad Fam. v. 12. 1).
'Rusticitas' often appears in our poet, most notably at iii. 127–8
'sed quia cultus adest, nec nostros mansit in annos / rusticitas
priscis illa superstes auis'. Applied to manners it conveys a lack
of polish, wit, and sophistication (the opposite of 'urbanitas')—
in dealings with the opposite sex, an inhibited awkwardness (672).

The term had a basis in fact, since remoter districts of Italy
preserved something of the old morality when it had all but
vanished from the capital (Tacitus, *Annals* xvi. 5. 1, cf. Virgil,
*Georgics* ii. 473–4). Ovid himself might have been expected to
show the qualities of his Paelignian ancestors; the juxtaposition
at *Amores* ii. 1. 1–2 strikes an almost defiant note, 'hoc quoque
composui Paelignis natus aquosis / ille ego nequitiae Naso poeta
meae.' But one should add that he thought it possible to show
*pudor* without being *rusticus* (cf. *Heroides* 20. 61 of Cydippe,
'uultus sine rusticitate pudentes').

**608. audentem Forsque Venusque iuuat :** adding Venus to the
well-known proverb (e.g. Terence, *Phormio* 203 'fortes Fortuna
adiuuat').

**609. non tua sub nostras ueniat facundia leges :** The didactic poet
may sometimes appeal to his reader and decline to go into
detail, as Lucretius v. 263, 1281–2 'nunc tibi quo pacto ferri
natura reperta / sit, facilest ipsi per te cognoscere, Memmi.'

**611–16.** Lines full of shrewd psychological insight, which reveal
this as a game of courtly love. 'You must play the lover' (611).
But are you not a real lover? This is always left obscure (cf.
439–40 'imitataque amantum / uerba'); the important thing is
credibility (*fides*, 612). And you should have no trouble here,
because every woman believes in her heart that she is beautiful
and adorable (613–14). Finally, however, a caution: at first you
may just go through the motions, but later find that you are
genuinely in love (615–16).

**614.** 'Every woman admires her own looks, however bad they may
be.'

**617–18.** An unexpected aside to the young women—Ovid only
starts to advise them in book iii. He assumes that a girl likes to
have admirers, preferably sincere but better insincere than none
at all. Therefore she should be kind to her suitor; even if he is
pretending at the moment, his love may soon become real.

**617. o :** The interjection adds a touch of solemnity (cf. Virgil,
*Georgics* ii. 35, quoted on 459).

**619. nunc sit :** 'Now should be the time.'

**620. ut pendens liquida ripa subestur aqua :** Axelson's emenda-
tion 'subestur' (*Hermes* 86 (1958), 127–8) is pointed to by the
manuscript readings and is undoubtedly right. It corresponds
exactly to ὑποτρώγων in Callimachus, *Ep.* 44 Pf. 3–4 πολλάκι λήθει /

τοῖχον ὑποτρώγων ἡσύχιος ποταμός—see further Nisbet and Hubbard on Horace, *Odes* i. 31. 8. For the illustration cf. 475–6 and Smith on Tibullus i. 4. 18.

**622. teretes digitos :** 'her well-proportioned fingers'. 'Teres' is defined by Festus as 'in longitudine rotundatum'; poets apply it to a neck, an arm, the calf of a leg. Munro (on Lucretius i. 35) writes that a *teres cervix* is a neck that has the true outline of beauty, neither lean nor fleshy, neither too long nor too short.

**623–6.** Another clever piece of psychology. Even chaste women like to have their beauty praised—witness the Judgement of Paris (625–6).

**626. nunc quoque :** for the mock aetiological style cf. 134. But why does Ovid say that Juno and Pallas *still* feel aggrieved over their failure to win the verdict? As to Pallas, I have no suggestion. Two possibilities spring to mind in the case of Juno. The goddess was believed to have nursed a long enmity towards the Roman people, partly due to the Judgement of Paris (cf. *Aeneid* i. 26–7 'manet alta mente repostum / iudicium Paridis spretaeque iniuria formae'). Alternatively, perhaps some ritual detail was thought to perpetuate Juno's anger at the judgement against her; thus in Nicander, *Alexipharmaca* 619 ff. (seemingly added lines) we are told that she will never accept a wreath of myrtle because Aphrodite wore one during the contest on Mount Ida.

**627. laudatas ostendit auis Iunonia pinnas :** The peacock was as much admired in ancient as in modern times for its spectacular beauty. It became the 'bird of Juno' because of its connection with her island of Samos (cf. Athenaeus xiv. 655a) and often figures on Samian coins. Ovid in the *Metamorphoses* tells how the hundred eyes of Argus were gathered into the peacock's tail (see Bömer on *Met.* i. 722). D'Arcy Thompson, *A Glossary of Greek Birds*, s.v. ταώς gives copious information on the bird in antiquity.

**laudatas :** the same doctrine in *Med. Fac.* 33, Pliny, *N.H.* x. 43 'gemmantes laudatus expandit colores', Dionysius, *de Auibus* i. 28 ('if anybody calls it beautiful').

**630. depexaeque iubae plausaque colla iuuant :** cf. *Georgics* iii. 185–6 (training horses for war or for racing) 'blandis gaudere magistri / laudibus et plausae sonitum ceruicis amare'.

**631–6.** *You can make any promise you like, adding an oath by any of the gods, because it is well established that lover's oath carries no penalty if false.*

**631. nec timide promitte : trahunt promissa puellas :** the antidote at iii. 461 'si bene promittent, totidem promittite uerbis.'

The lover's oath became a notorious commonplace (for its origin, see on 635–6 below). But Ovid follows in particular

Tibullus i. 4. 21–6 (K. F. Smith ad loc. collects many other parallels):

> nec iurare time: Veneris periuria uenti
> irrita per terras et freta summa ferunt.
> gratia magna Ioui: uetuit pater ipse ualere
> iurasset cupide quidquid ineptus amor;
> perque suas impune sinit Dictynna sagittas
> adfirmes, crines perque Minerua suos.

**634. Aeolios . . . Notos :** Aeolus was entrusted with the guardian-ship of all the winds (e.g. *Aeneid* i. 52 ff.).

**635–6. per Styga Iunoni falsum iurare solebat / Iuppiter : exemplo nunc fauet ipse suo :** The dispensation was held to derive from Zeus' affair with Io; he swore falsely to Hera that he had not touched the girl, and thereafter ordained that the oaths of mortals in love should carry no penalty, ἐκ τοῦ δ' ὅρκον ἔθηκεν ἀποί-νιμον ἀνθρώποισι / νοσφιδίων ἔργων πέρι Κύπριδος (Pseudo-Hesiod fr. 124 Merkelbach–West).

**635. per Styga :** the most awesome oath amongst the gods (*Iliad* xv. 37–8)—this touch looks like an Ovidian refinement.

**636. exemplo nunc fauet ipse suo :** a motif very common in Greek epigram (see on 526).

**637–44.** *Do not imagine that you can swear by the gods so lightly over any other matter. We must believe in their existence, power, and concern for human conduct, in order to reinforce our moral laws. Observe all your proper obligations ; only in this sphere may you deceive.*

A very well-known passage (discussed by Wilkinson, *Ovid Recalled*, p. 191, Fränkel, *Ovid, a Poet between Two Worlds*, p. 90, Brooks Otis, *TAPA* 1938, 209–10). Perhaps the most valuable question to ask is: what reaction did Ovid expect from his first audience to these lines? It has been almost universally assumed that the poet intended to provoke and shock, but this verdict has to a great extent derived from quoting the lines (particularly 637) out of context, and seems at least disputable. To me the surprising point is rather that he thought fit to insert a weighty passage in such a frivolous context; one might have imagined the lover's oath to be so well-worn a topic as to need neither explanation nor apology.

How much of Ovid's personal *credo* should we see here? Of course this is difficult to tell, particularly in a work which is for the most part a *jeu d'esprit*. But if he was sceptical about the existence of the Olympian gods while holding at the same time that belief in them (together with the maintenance of long-standing religious ceremonies) helped social morality, many of his countrymen at the time must have agreed with him.

**637-40.** Servius (on *Aeneid* iv. 379) conveniently summarizes the three main opinions held about the gods: 'deos non esse . . . esse et nihil curare, ut Epicurei, esse et curare, ut Stoici'. In 637 Ovid rejects the first view (though hardly in a manner to satisfy a theist), and in 639-40 the second. As a commentary on these lines it is worth reading Cicero, *de Natura Deorum* i. 61 ff. with Pease's notes.

**637. expedit esse deos :** probably going back to an anecdote told of Diogenes, who, when asked whether the gods existed, replied that he did not know but thought it expedient that they should (Tertullian, *ad Nationes* ii. 2). A famous tragic fragment, ascribed alternatively to Critias (fr. 1 *T.G.F.*²) or to Euripides, goes further—men deliberately invented the gods as a deterrent to wrongdoing.

**638. dentur in antiquos tura merumque focos :** suggesting the ordered ritual of the Roman state. Ovid here is not so far from the pragmatism of Cicero: 'nam et maiorum instituta tueri sacris caerimoniisque retinendis sapientis est' (*de Div.* ii. 148, cf. Pease on *de Natura Deorum* i. 61 'caerimonias . . . tuendas').

**639-40.** This couplet is directed against the Epicurean conception of the gods as remote beings who have no interest in human affairs, and certainly do not punish sin. Epicurus himself wrote that wrongdoing should be avoided just because the fear of detection by human agency destroyed peace of mind. Not surprisingly he suffered heavy criticism on this point (Usener, *Epicurea*, frs. 531-4).

**639. secura quies :** Both 'securus' and 'quies' ('quietus') recur in Epicurean descriptions of the gods; compare Lucretius v. 82 'nam bene qui didicere deos securum agere aeuum' (picked up by Horace, *Sat.* i. 5. 101), and their 'sedes quietae' at Lucretius iii. 18 ff. (also Pease on *Aeneid* iv. 379-80 'ea cura quietos / sollicitat').

**similisque sopori :** While Epicureans might enthuse over the blessed tranquillity which they provided for their gods, opponents of the sect were more likely to draw a picture of sloth and idleness, e.g. Tertullian, *Apol.* 47. 6 'Epicurei (*sc.* deum adseuerant) otiosum et inexercitum' (more material in Usener, *Epicurea*, pp. 241-4). Earlier Plato had been no less scornful of any such doctrine (*Laws* x. 900-1).

**640. numen adest :** As Wilkinson notes (p. 191), not necessarily a statement of Ovid's own belief, but rather what Roman parents should teach their children. The words could almost be in inverted commas.

**641-2. reddite depositum ; pietas sua foedera seruet ; / fraus absit ; uacuas caedis habete manus :** Here in outline we may recognize a pagan counterpart to the Jewish commandments (cf. also

*Amores* iii. 9. 37 'uiue pius . . . pius cole sacra'). From the fifth
century B.C. Greek literature offers a small body of ordinances
(usually three) sometimes called the 'unwritten laws'. The first
two are invariably 'Worship the gods' and 'Honour your
parents'; the third may be 'Do not swear a false oath', 'Obey
the laws' or 'Respect the stranger'. See the Headlam–Thomson
edition of Aeschylus, *The Oresteia* on *Eumenides* 269–72. Among
fuller collections one can cite the Delphic precepts, the Golden
Sayings ascribed to Pythagoras, and the *Sententiae* of Pseudo-
Phocylides (late, since they show influence from the New as well
as the Old Testament); these last two appear with notes in the
Teubner *Theognis* (ed. Douglas Young). In a Roman milieu
there were 'Sayings of Cato' current at least by the time of
Plutarch; the surviving *Disticha Catonis* (not of course from
the Elder Cato himself) as prefaced by a later catalogue which
starts 'Deo supplica, parentes ama, cognatos cole, datum serua'
(Baehrens, *P.L.M.* III, p. 214). It seems reasonable to conclude
that Ovid would have known more than one such collection,
possibly in verse.

**641. reddite depositum :** This may surprise us as a primary obli-
gation. But before the days of safe deposit in a bank, people
would leave valuable property with a friend, and to return it on
demand was a sacred duty (cf. Juvenal, 13. 15–16 'sacrum tibi
quod non reddat amicus / depositum'). When the younger Pliny
investigated the worship of Christians in his province, he found
that their oath, derived in the main from the Ten Command-
ments (but see Sherwin-White ad loc.) included the promise 'ne
depositum adpellati abnegarent' (*Epist.* x. 96. 7). Finally, three
variations on the theme: (a) the story of Glaucus, whose family
was blotted out because he merely considered not returning
a deposit (Herodotus vi. 86), (b) the discussion of virtue defined
as 'rendering to each man his due' is conducted partly in terms
of returning things deposited (Plato, *Republic* i. 331e3 ff., cf.
Cicero, *de Officiis* iii. 95), (c) a lady who had broken all the rules,
'saepe antehac fidem prodiderat, *creditum abiurauerat*, caedis
conscia fuerat' (Sallust, *Catiline* 25).

**pietas sua foedera seruet :** particularly the duty to one's
parents (see above).

**642.** These two prohibitions are linked in Pseudo-Phocylides line
4 μήτε δόλους ῥάπτειν μήθ' αἵματι χεῖρα μιαίνειν.

**643. si sapitis :** 'take my advice', a colloquial admonitory touch,
as e.g. *Met.* xiv. 675 (on this and similar phrases, see J. B.
Hofmann, *Lateinische Umgangssprache*[2], pp. 134 and 200).

**644.** †hac magis est una fraude pudenda fides† : I believe with
Goold (*Harvard Studies* 69 (1965), 41) and others that the
solution to this crux lies in 'hac *minus* est una fraude *tuenda*

fides', 'with the exception of this one deceit good faith should be kept' (for *minus*+abl. = except for cf. *Met.* xii. 554 'me minus uno').

Naugerius claimed to have found 'tuenda' 'in nonnullis', and Heinsius recorded it from an unidentified manuscript. Burman, taking up Naugerius, interpreted the line with 'minus' and 'tuenda'; Kenney himself favoured this solution, but not to the extent of printing it in his Oxford Text. For manuscript confusion between 'minus' and 'magis' cf. *Heroides* 17. 104; quite often we find a word corrupted into its opposite (see Housman on Manilius v. 463).

**645–58.** *Furthermore women are for the most part perjured, and it is an age-old saying that inventors of evil deserve to perish by their own devices. Witness the stories of Busiris and Phalaris.*

**646. in laqueos, quos posuere, cadant :** proverbial (see Otto *s.v. Laqueus* 1).

**647–56.** These lines make an interesting piece of literary history involving the *Aetia* of Callimachus (see Appendix IV), and serve to illustrate Ovid's wide knowledge and use of the Hellenistic poets. We can just pick up his allusion because of the fragmentary state of the *Aetia*; there must be many similar instances as yet undetected. The closely parallel passage in Claudian (*in Eutropium* i. 157–66) may depend on Ovid rather than Callimachus:

> quam bene dispositum terris, ut dignus iniqui
> fructus consilii primis auctoribus instet.
> sic multos fluuio uates arente per annos
> hospite qui caeso monuit placare Tonantem,
> inuentas primus Busiridis imbuit aras
> et cecidit saeui, quod dixerat, hostia sacri.
> sic opifex tauri tormentorumque repertor,
> qui funesta nouo fabricauerat aera dolori,
> primus inexpertum Siculo cogente tyranno
> sensit opus docuitque suum mugire iuuencum.

**647–52.** Busiris was a mythical king of Egypt (in fact 'Busiris' means 'House of Osiris', and was the name of more than one Egyptian town), appearing first in Pherecydes. After the incident described here he tried to repeat the operation when visited by Heracles—not surprisingly he found that he had caught a Tartar! Although the king himself is mythical, the legend may preserve distant memories of human sacrifice in Egypt at a very early date to ensure the rising of the Nile (see How and Wells on Herodotus ii. 45).

**647–8. iuuantibus arua / imbribus :** Ovid must have known that Egypt depended on the Nile flood, not on rainfall; to quote Seneca 'aut nulli imbres sunt, aut rari et qui insuetam aquis

caelestibus terram non adiuuent' (*Q.N.* iv. a.2). Either, then, he
is championing a theory which ascribed the flood to rain near
the Nile's source, or 'imbres' are themselves the flood-waters of
the river. In two papyri quoted by LSJ ὄμβρος is used of the Nile's
inundation; also in a poetic piece (Kenyon, *Rev. de Phil.* 19
(1895), 177 ff. line 11) ἐλευθερίου Διὸς ὄμβρον.

**649. Thrasius :** a seer said to have come from Cyprus.

**650. adfuso :** almost a technical term of sacrifice (cf. *Fasti* i. 360).

**651–2.** Zeus is normally the protector of strangers, so in a sense
Thrasius deserved his fate.

**653–4.** Unlike Busiris, Phalaris was a real enough character,
tyrant of Acragas in Sicily *c.* 570–554 B.C. and notorious for his
cruelty. The historian Timaeus, himself a Sicilian, said some-
thing about the bull, but no extant authority before Calli-
machus recalls the fate of its inventor. After the tyrant's death
his subjects threw the bull into the sea; a scholiast on Pindar,
*Pythian* i. 185 adds that what tourists were shown as the bull of
Phalaris was really a figure of the bull-headed river god Gela.

**653. uiolenti . . . Perilli :** 'a good craftsman but a bad man'
(Lucian, *Phalaris* I. 11), cf. Propertius ii. 25. 12 'et gemere in
tauro, saeue Perille, tuo'. Perillus is a diminutive form of the
name Perilaus.

**654. inbuit :** basically 'to dip', thence to use for the first time or
'inaugurate' (cf. the English 'house-warming party'); the verb
corresponds exactly to ἐκαίνισεν in Callimachus fr. 46. 1 (Appen-
dix IV). *Tristia* iii. 11. 45 ff. describes the handing-over cere-
mony: '"adspicis a dextra latus hoc adapertile tauri? / hac
tibi, quem perdes, coniciendus erit. / protinus inclusum lentis
carbonibus ure: / mugiet, et ueri uox erit illa bouis. / pro quibus
inuentis, ut munus munere penses, / da, precor, ingenio praemia
digna meo." / dixerat, at Phalaris "poenae mirande repertor, /
ipse tuum praesens imbue" dixit "opus!"'

**655. iustus uterque fuit :** something of a paradox, because in
general both were famed for injustice (cf. Virgil, *Georgics* iii. 5
'inlaudati . . . Busiridis'). The encomia of Busiris by Polycrates
and Isocrates were demonstrations of how rhetoric could make
the worse cause the better. As for Phalaris, the common opinion
was that he performed his sole just act in killing Perillus.

   **neque enim lex aequior ulla est :** the *lex talionis*, or, as the
Greeks put it, εἴ κε πάθοι τά τ' ἔρεξε, δίκη κ' ἰθεῖα γένοιτο ('if a man
were to suffer what he did, then true justice would be done',
ps.-Hesiod fr. 286 M–W). In the (? 2nd cent. A.D.) 'Epistles of
Phalaris' 122. 3 the king is made to say, perhaps echoing Calli-
machus, 'I am convinced that no one among you or the rest of
the Greeks will think it unjust that an inventor of an outrage for
others should have his fill of it himself.'

**659-68.** *Together with your promises you should bring tears to play on her, and kisses amid your flattery.*

**659. et lacrimae prosunt :** For the didactic touch see on 159, and for the utility of tears Propertius i. 12. 15–16 'felix qui potuit praesenti flere puellae: / non nihil aspersis gaudet Amor lacrimis' with K. F. Smith on Tibullus i. 4. 71–2.

    **lacrimis adamanta mouebis :** cf. Theocritus 2. 33–4 τὺ δ' Ἄρτεμι καὶ τὸν ἐν Ἄιδα / κινήσαις ἀδάμαντα, Otto, *Sprichwörter*, s.v. Adamas. 'Adamant' refers first to any hard metal, then to the diamond. Symbolically it represents anything immutable and inexorable; in particular the gates of the Underworld are made of adamant (Gow on Theocritus 2. 33–4, cf. Propertius iv. 11. 4 'non exorato stant adamante uiae').

**661-2.** False tears—for this topic compare *Amores* i. 8. 83–4 'quin etiam discant oculi lacrimare coacti, / et faciant udas ille uel ille genas', *Heroides* 2. 51–2 (Phyllis to Demophoon) 'credidimus lacrimis: an et hae simulare docentur? / hae quoque habent artes, quaque iubentur eunt?', Juvenal 6. 273–5, Martial i. 33.

**662. uncta . . . manu :** The manuscript evidence undoubtedly points to *uncta* rather than *uda* (though Y has 'uda'). Kenney wonders whether ancient ointments would contain something pungent so as to produce the effect of tears. But may we not widen the application of 'uncta' to include anything greasy? To quote *The Taming of the Shrew*: 'And if the boy have not a woman's gift / To rain a shower of commanded tears, / An onion will do well for such a shift, / Which in a napkin being close conveyed / Shall in despite enforce a watery eye.'

**665-6.** See on 127.

**667-8.** Paul Turner remarks that Dryden here makes Ovid sound like an advertisement for razor-blades: 'Kiss only soft, I charge you, and forbear / With your hard bristles not to brush the fair.'

**669-80.** *After kissing her you would be foolish not to go the whole way. You may have inhibitions about using 'force', but that kind of force need not be unwelcome to its victim.*

**671.** 'How much was there between kissing her and the completion of your desire?' For *deesse*+dative cf. 177–8.

**672. ei mihi :** This interjection, frequent in early Comedy and occasionally found in Epic and Tragedy, is much used by Ovid (e.g. 741); see Austin on *Aeneid* ii. 274.

    **rusticitas, non pudor ille fuit :** For the terms, see on 607–8. But here 'pudor' is what the hesitater cites in his own defence (i.e. an admirable quality), while 'rusticitas' views the same conduct from a different angle.

**674. inuitae saepe dedisse uolunt :** characteristically Ovidian— they may not wish *dare*, but are glad *dedisse*, cf. *Amores* iii. 11. 4

'et quae non puduit ferre, tulisse pudet' (picked up by Seneca, *Epist.* 78. 14 'quod acerbum fuit ferre, tulisse iucundum est').

**678. ut simulet uultu gaudia :** 'even supposing she pretends to look happy'. Contrast the girl in Theocritus 27. 70, who, after making secret love, leaves ὄμμασιν αἰδομένοις, κραδίη δέ οἱ ἔνδον ἰάνθη.

**679–80.** Castor and Pollux were said to have abstracted by force Phoebe and Hilaira, the daughters of Leucippus (Prop. i. 2. 15–16), who were engaged to Lynceus and Idas (*Fasti* v. 699 ff., Theocritus 22. 137 ff.). The preference of the young ladies (680) is not recorded elsewhere; often the ensuing fight resulted in Castor's death.

**681–704.** The point is made at length by the legend of Achilles and Deidamia. At the beginning of the Trojan war Thetis, the divine mother of Achilles, realized that her son would die if he went to Troy and therefore concealed him on the island of Scyros, disguised as a girl. There, however, he fell in love with the princess Deidamia, daughter of Lycomedes, and she bore to him Neoptolemus or Pyrrhus. This story was the subject of Euripides' *Scyrians* (Webster, *The Tragedies of Euripides*, pp. 95–7)—the *Scyrians* of Sophocles may have treated a different episode. One Euripidean fragment (880 *T.G.F.*²), unplaced but plausibly assigned to the *Scyrians*, resembles Ovid lines 691–6: οὐκ ἐν γυναιξὶ τοὺς νεανίας χρεών / ἀλλ' ἐν σιδήρῳ κἂν ὅπλοις τιμὰς ἔχειν ('young men should win honour in arms and warfare, not in the company of women'). For the myth in the fifth century and earlier see also O. A. W. Dilke's edition of Statius, *Achilleid*, pp. 11–12.

But the immediate source for our poet was clearly the so-called *Epithalamium of Achilles and Deidamia*, sometimes, though hazardously, attributed to Bion, who flourished *c.* 100 B.C. (piece 2 of Pseudo-Bion in Gow's *Bucolici Graeci*, parts reproduced and translated in my Appendix V); we have 32 lines of the poem before the manuscripts break off. Since the authorship is in fact quite uncertain, we see Ovid using a very recherché bit of Hellenistic poetry. The result, however, is not one of his happiest creations; one misses the sparkle which characterizes most digressions in the *Ars*, and to me at least the rhetorical antitheses of 691–6 become wearisome. From later literature the treatment in Statius, *Achilleid* i shows many points of contact with Ovid.

**681. fabula nota quidem, sed non indigna referri :** for such feigned indifference cf. *Fasti* iv. 417–18 'exigit ipse locus raptus ut uirginis edam: / plura recognosces, pauca docendus eris.' The technique seems Callimachean (cf. 297)—one is reminded of the way Callimachus, before launching into the story of the blind-

ing of Tiresias, adds μῦθος δ' οὐκ ἐμός, ἀλλ' ἑτέρων (*hymn* 5. 56 'the
tale is not mine, but comes from others').

**682. Haemonio :** 'Thessalian'.

**683-90.** A lightning summary of previous events, written in such
a way that it assumes knowledge of the story on the part of
readers—note the elliptical references to the Judgement of
Paris (683-4) and the anger of Menelaus (687-8) with no names
given. All this is typical of Hellenistic poetry. No doubt Ovid
bases himself on lines 10-15 of the *Epithalamium* (Appendix V);
other passages showing similar technique are Theocritus 22.
27 ff. (cf. the opening of Catullus 64 and Propertius i. 20. 17-20)
and the prologue to Apollonius' *Argonautica* (i. 5-17).

**683. mala praemia :** In return for his vote Aphrodite granted
Paris the winning of Helen.

**684. uincere digna duas :** cf. *Heroides* 16. 70 'uincere quae forma
digna sit una duas'. The phrase is given some edge by its pro-
verbial quality (as e.g. Plato, *Phaedo* 89c πρὸς δύο λέγεται οὐδ'
ὁ 'Ηρακλῆς οἷός τε εἶναι, Catullus 62. 64 'noli pugnare duobus').

**685. diuerso . . . orbe :** cf. *Aeneid* vii. 223-4 'quibus actus uterque /
Europae atque Asiae fatis concurrerit orbis' (that the Trojan
war was a struggle between two continents became a common-
place, e.g. Catullus 68. 89). But to catch the essence of the
phrase is not easy. 'From a different world' over-dramatizes it,
while 'from another continent' misses the idea of being enclosed
and spiritually separate. The exiled Ovid felt that he was
writing 'diuersum . . . in orbem' (*ex Ponto* i. 5. 67) from his own
position 'Scythico . . . in orbe' (*Tristia* iii. 12. 51); a citizen of
the empire might speak of 'noster orbis'. See Joseph Vogt,
*Orbis Romanus* (1929), pp. 23-6. In English 'the New World' has
about the same tone.

**687. iurabant omnes in laesi uerba mariti :** Before setting out from
Aulis the Greeks swore not to return until they had sacked Troy
(*Iliad* ii. 286 ff.); contrast *Aeneid* iv. 425-6 of Dido 'non ego
cum Danais Troianam exscindere gentem / Aulide iuraui.'
    **iurabant . . . in . . . uerba :** Properly this means swearing in
words dictated by the man who administers the oath. A Roman
soldier at the beginning of each campaign would bind himself
with the *sacramentum* of loyalty to his commander; so, ac-
cording to Augustus, did the whole of Italy before Actium,
'iurauit in mea uerba tota Italia' (*Res Gestae* 25. 2).

**688. publica causa :** 'a national cause', cf. Livy ii. 56 'post publi-
cam causam priuato dolore habito'.

**689.** Achilles' acquiescence would have been disgraceful had it
not been prompted by *pietas* towards his mother Thetis.

**690. ueste uirum longa dissimulatus erat :** from line 7 of the
*Epithalamium* πῶς παῖς ἔσσατο φᾶρος, ὅπως δ' ἐψεύσατο μορφάν, 'how

the boy put on a girl's dress and disguised his appearance' (for the contrast between Achilles and the other Greeks cf. also *Epithalamium* 15).

**691–6.** Characteristic lines, but somewhat irritating. He has taken one rather obvious antithesis, which appears also in the *Epithalamium* (16 εἴρια δ᾽ ἀνθ᾽ ὅπλων ἐδιδάσκετο), and produced a fourfold amplification (691–2, 693, 694, 695–6). Surely we see here the *bad* influence of rhetoric on Ovid's style.

**691. quid facis, Aeacide?** : apostrophizing him in the same way as he does Pasiphae (303 ff.). The epic-style patronymic (in fact Achilles was grandson of Aeacus) heightens the contrast between his present occupation and the one proper to him.

**692. alia Palladis arte** : 'by a different accomplishment of Pallas'. Athena, besides being the patron of spinning (cf. her contest with Arachne at *Met.* vi. 1 ff.), was a warrior goddess (*Met.* viii. .264 'bellatricemque Mineruam').

**693 ff.** These lines contain a number of references to the technique of spinning; for a useful account of the whole process (with illustrations), see R. J. Forbes, *Studies in Ancient Technology*, vol. IV, (ed. 2, Leiden, 1964), pp. 149 ff., and for a full poetic description Catullus 64. 311 ff.

**693. quid tibi cum calathis?** : The baskets would hold wool which had been washed and carded but still awaited spinning.

**694. pensa** : the amount given to a girl for her daily task (from *pendo*, literally 'what is weighed out').

**in dextra, qua cadet Hector** : for Achilles' hands, see on 15–16.

**695. reice succinctos operoso stamine fusos** : 'Lay aside the spindles covered with worked thread.' After being washed and carded, the wool had its fibres arranged lengthways by an instrument called the *epinetrum*, and then was placed on the distaff (*colus*, 702), which the spinner stuck under her left arm or in her girdle, to leave both hands free. The left hand held the spindle, while the right drew wool from the distaff, attaching the thread to the stem of the spindle, and then turned the spindle (aided by a whorl at its end) with thumb and forefinger.

**succinctos** : perhaps humorous—the threads form a kind of short skirt on the spindle.

**696. quassanda est ista Pelias hasta manu** : Only Achilles could brandish his great spear, the Πηλιὰς μελίη, so called because it was cut from Mt. Pelion; cf. *Iliad* xvi. 141–3 τὸ μὲν οὐ δύνατ᾽ ἄλλος Ἀχαιῶν / πάλλειν, ἀλλά μιν οἶος ἐπίστατο πῆλαι Ἀχιλλεύς / Πηλιάδα μελίην. Homer obviously is making a play between Πηλιάς and πῆλαι, which *quassanda* reflects in Ovid.

**698.** cf. *Epithalamium* 21 θυμὸν δ᾽ ἀνέρος εἶχε καὶ ἀνέρος εἶχεν ἔρωτα, Statius, *Ach.* i. 561–2 and 639 (Achilles to himself) 'teque marem (pudet heu!) nec amore probabis?'

**699. uiribus illa quidem uicta est (ita credere oportet) :** The parenthesis shows his dependence on literary tradition in the learned Hellenistic manner (see Fordyce on Catullus 64. 1–2) and adds the implication 'though we might prefer to think it was by consent'. Similarly Statius, *Ach*. i. 642 'ui potitur uotis.

**700. sed uoluit uinci uiribus illa tamen :** the repetition of words emphasizing 'uoluit' (within increased alliteration). Such repetition is a striking feature of our poet's style, often combined with a reversal of word-order (uiribus . . . uicta est—uinci uiribus). Compare 191–2 'auspiciis annisque—annis auspiciisque', *Met*. i. 590–1 ' "pete" dixerat "*umbras* / altorum *nemorum*" (et *nemorum* monstrauerat *umbras*) ', viii. 860 '*litore* in hoc *steterat* (nam *stantem* in *litore* uidi).'

**701. saepe 'mane' dixit, cum iam properaret Achilles :** Attempts to delay the traveller and reproaches for his cruelty in leaving are common in a *propempticon* (Cairns, *Generic Composition*, p. 138 etc.). True to type, Statius gives Deidamia a long speech (*Ach*. i. 929 ff.)—'cara ceruice mariti / fusa noui lacrimas iam soluit et occupat artus : / "adspiciamne iterum meque hoc in pectore ponam?" ' (and so on for 25 lines).

**702. fortia . . . arma :** The epithet contributes something, because spinning implements might themselves be termed 'arma' of a different kind (cf. Virgil, *Georgics* i. 160 'duris agrestibus arma' of farming tools, Martial xiv. 36. 1 'tondendis haec arma tibi sunt apta capillis'). Achilles was tricked into revealing himself by picking up martial weapons at the sound of a trumpet (Statius, *Ach*. i. 878 ff., cf. 'sumpserat' here).

**703. uis ubi nunc illa est? :** for the mocking or indignant question cf. Tibullus ii. 3. 27 'Delos ubi nunc, Phoebe, tua est, ubi Delphica Pytho?' (in Greek ποῦ may be used similarly).

**705–14.** Drawing the moral from the preceding story : *a man must always take the initiative and not wait to be asked*. For a woman to make the first move was generally thought to be the height of shamelessness, e.g. *Amores* i. 8. 43–4 (in the mouth of the horrible old woman Dipsas, and arousing the indignation of her hearer (109 ff.)) 'casta est quam nemo rogauit; / aut, si rusticitas non uetat, ipsa rogat', Sallust, *Catiline* 25 'lubido sic adcensa ut saepius peteret uiros quam peteretur'.

**709–10.** The proper way in which a love affair should be conducted, with due respect to the decencies on both sides.

**710. comiter :** 'graciously', with relaxed encouragement. Compare Tacitus, *Ann*. v. 1 on Livia 'comis ultra quam antiquis feminis probatum', and contrast the abrupt and alarming manners of Tiberius 'non . . . comi uia sed horridus ac plerumque formidatus' (*Ann*. iv. 7).

**712.** 'Take the first step to bring about your desire.'

**714.** Of course the idea of any of the mythical heroines trying to seduce Jupiter is intentionally ridiculous.

**715. tumidos accedere fastus :** Her scorn is aroused by the lover's grovelling and too insistent prayers. Kenney earlier gave serious consideration to the better-attested variant 'abscedere' printed by Lenz, which can mean to depart (of feelings or emotions e.g. aegritudo, nausea, lubido). Ovid would then be recommending the young man to ease up as soon as he feels that his entreaties have begun to break down her resistance, in order to excite her interest even more (717). That is shrewd psychology, closely resembling the advice at ii. 349 ff. 'cum tibi maior erit fiducia, posse requiri, / cum procul absenti cura futurus eris,/ da requiem.' But at this stage of the affair the lover has not yet a firm enough hold on his lady's affection, and should press home every advantage. So Kenney was probably right to reject 'abscedere' in the last analysis (*CQ* 1962, 20 n. 1).

**717. quod refugit, multae cupiunt ; odere, quod instat :** a famous *topos*, which goes back to Sappho (191. 21 ff. *Lyrica Graeca Selecta*) καὶ γὰρ αἰ φεύγει, ταχέως διώξει· / αἰ δὲ δῶρα μὴ δέκετ', ἀλλὰ δώσει· / αἰ δὲ μὴ φίλει, ταχέως φιλήσει / κωὐκ ἐθέλοισα (κωῦ σε θέλοισαν Knox), 'for if she flees, she will soon pursue; and if she receives not gifts, yet shall she give; and if she loves not, she shall soon love, even against her will' (or 'even when you would not') as translated by Page (*Sappho and Alcaeus*, p. 4). Hellenistic poets took up the idea, e.g. Theocritus on Galatea (6. 17) καὶ φεύγει φιλέοντα καὶ οὐ φιλέοντα διώκει, and Callimachus, *Ep.* 31. For more material see Nisbet and Hubbard's Introduction to Horace, *Odes* i. 33.

**719–22.** An even more indirect approach—*pretend to be just a good friend*.

**721. uidi :** the insistence upon personal experience proper to a didactic poet (see Kenney in *Ovidiana*, p. 202, adding e.g. [Oppian], *Cyn.* iii. 482 ναὶ μὴν ἄλλο γένεθλον ἐμοῖς ἴδον ὀφθαλμοῖσιν).

**tetricae . . . puellae :** a girl who professed the rigid, old-fashioned morality associated particularly with the Sabines, to whom this epithet is often applied (*Amores* iii. 8. 61, Livy, i. 18. 4). In fact there was a mountain called Tetrica or Tetricus in the territory of the Sabines, which seemed to reflect their character (cf. *Aeneid* vii. 713–14 'qui Tetricae horrentis rupes montemque Seuerum / Casperiamque colunt').

**data uerba :** in the phrase 'dare uerba' = to cheat or deceive, the essence of uerba is 'mere empty words'.

**722. cultor :** 'a devoted attendant'. Cicero (*ad Att.* x. 8. 9) thanks Atticus for kindness shown to his daughter, 'meam Tulliam suauissime diligentissimeque coluisti'; similarly Aeneas with Dido's sister 'solam nam perfidus ille / te colere' (*Aen.* iv. 421–2).

**723 ff.** At this point the argument of bk. i is complete—the girl
has been found and caught. We end with a number of miscel-
laneous precepts which are made to seem afterthoughts (par-
ticularly 755 'finiturus eram').

**723–38.** *A lover, unlike a sailor, farmer, or athlete, should be pale,
thin, and sickly-looking.* Matters of dress and personal appear-
ance have been dealt with earlier (505 ff.); while Ovid there
reflected more robust Roman ideals, the present lines are com-
pletely within the tradition of love-poetry.

**723. candidus in nauta turpis color :** Although Romans might
admire a fair complexion in men as a sign of free-birth (*ingenuus
color* as opposed to *color seruilis*, see Shackleton Bailey on Pro-
pertius i. 4. 13), a lack of sunburn was usually thought repre-
hensible, as suggested by 513 'fuscentur corpora Campo'—and
so with the Greeks, e.g. Euripides, *Bacchae* 457–8 λευκὴν δὲ χροιὰν
ἐκ παρασκευῆς ἔχεις / οὐχ ἡλίου βολαῖσιν, ἀλλ' ὑπὸ σκιᾶς. The surprising
point is that 'candidus . . . color' here by implication is equated
with the lover's *pallor* in 729. Normally 'candidus' denotes a
brilliant white, while 'albus' (a dead white) can be a more sickly
hue ('albus pallor' at Horace, *Epodes* 7. 15), but we sometimes
find 'candidus' taking over the associations of 'albus' (see J.
André, *Études sur les termes de couleur dans la langue latine*
(1949), pp. 33–5).

**724. sideris :** 'the sun'. For this usage, see Bömer on *Met.* i. 779.

**725. turpis et agricolae :** sc. candidus color.

**726. sub Ioue :** 'under the open sky'.

**727. Palladiae petitur cui fama coronae :** the Olympic athlete, who
competed for the prize of an olive garland (the olive being sacred
to Pallas). Although the prestige of the Games had declined by
Ovid's day, the Olympic competitor had a place in the tradi-
tional *topos* cataloguing and comparing different occupations
(see Nisbet and Hubbard's Introduction to Horace, *Odes* i. 1 and
on i. 1. 3)—a list into which our poet has incongruously slipped
the lover.

**729. palleat omnis amans :** perhaps the most notorious sign of love,
going back in Greek poetry to Sappho 199. 14–15 *Lyrica Graeca
Selecta* χλωροτέρα δὲ ποίας / ἔμμι ('I am paler than grass'). Many
more instances (among them Theocritus 2. 88, Catullus 64. 100)
are collected by Rohde, *Der Griechische Roman*[3], p. 157 n. 2.
Fordyce (on Catullus 81. 4) points out that the shade denoted by
'pallere' includes a yellowish tinge, appropriate to the Mediter-
ranean complexion.

**730. hoc decet, hoc †multi non ualuisse putant† :** The general sense
is clear enough—paleness in a lover is both *decorum* and *utile*—
but restoration has caused much trouble (I extend the *cruces*
in Kenney's OCT, since 'multi' and 'putant' are open to

suspicion, though 'non ualuisse' may well be sound). Palmer
suggested 'multis non ualuisse putas?', Kenney 'multis mox
ualuisse putant'. Against the latter Goold (*Harvard Studies* 69
(1965), 67) objected that the logic 'let *every* lover pale; it has
done the trick for *many*' carries the damaging implication that
for some the precept has proved unsuccessful—rather pedanti-
cally, but the conjecture does not appeal to me. Goold himself
favoured 'hoc stulti ('only fools') non ualuisse putant' (Hertz-
berg), which Kenney rightly described as 'somewhat inurbane'.
   I propose 'hoc nulli (dative singular) non ualuisse puta',
'consider that this has proved effective for all' (followed by the
example of two unlikely characters whom pallor helped). For
'nulli non' placed thus in a pentameter cf. 614. In fact 'nulli'
was suggested by Mueller, but as nominative plural with
'putent'; a misunderstanding over the case could have contri-
buted to the original corruption of 'puta'.

**731–2.** Orion the great hunter and Daphnis the shepherd might be
expected to have a sunburned complexion (cf. 723 ff.), but in
love they found pallor beneficial. The two legends referred to are
exceedingly obscure (probably from lost Alexandrian poetic
sources) and we can only guess at their details; the point, how-
ever, must be that both Orion and Daphnis were eventually
successful in their suit.

**731. pallidus in Side siluis errabat Orion :** Side (if correctly re-
stored by Schulze) was the first wife of Orion, cast into Hades
because she rivalled Hera in beauty (Apollodorus i. 4. 3).
Kenney offered an ingenious explanation for the confused manu-
script readings: according to Philargyrius on Virgil, *Ecl.* 5. 20
the nymph to whom *Daphnis* swore constancy was Lyca, so
'Lyca' may have been added as a gloss to 'Naide' in 732, dis-
placing a proper name in the line above and becoming corrupted
itself through Orion's well-known habit of hunting lynxes.

   **pallidus in Side :** 'in' means 'over', 'in the case of'. We often
find 'ardeo in'+ablative (e.g. *Met.* viii. 50, cf. Callimachus fr.
67. 2 $\mathring{\eta}\theta\epsilon\tau o \ldots \epsilon\pi\iota$), and the construction is extended to other
words or phrases—cf. *Amores* iii. 6. 25–6 'Inachus in Melie
Bithynide pallidus isse / dicitur', Catullus 64. 98 'in flauo saepe
hospite suspirantem'.

   **siluis errabat Orion :** following his normal occupation, but in
a distraught condition (cf. Orion in a different context at
Cicero, *Aratea* fr. 33. 421–4 'excelsis errans in collibus amens . . . /
ille feras uaecors amenti corde necabat'). Kenney wonders
whether he is hunting to furnish a bride-price, as for another lady
in Parthenius, *Narr. Amat.* 20. Even for those not that way
inclined, hunting regularly provides a distraction from un-
happy love, e.g. Virgil, *Ecl.* 10. 52–3 (Gallus) 'certum est in

siluis inter spelaea ferarum / malle pati', Propertius i. 1. 11–12
'nam modo Partheniis amens errabat in antris, / ibat et hir-
sutas ille uidere feras' (Milanion has the added advantage that
he can be near his beloved Atalanta).

732. **pallidus in lenta Naide Daphnis erat** : For the multifarious
legend of Daphnis see Gow's introduction to Theocritus 1; here
we want a story in which he overcomes the previous reluctance
of his love. The mention of Nais (which may mean 'a water-
nymph' or be a proper name) points to Theocritus 8. 93 καὶ
νύμφαν ἄκραβος ἐὼν ἔτι Ναΐδα γᾶμεν where, however, nothing is said of
any earlier rebuff. In Theocritus 7. 73 ff. Daphnis is rejected by
Xenea, and in Nonnus xv. 308 ff. by an unnamed nymph.

733. **arguat et macies animum** : second only to pallor as an indi-
cation of love, cf. Theocritus 2. 88–90, *Amores* ii. 9. 14, and a
characteristic variation at *Amores* i. 6. 3–6 where Ovid tells the
surly *ostiarius* that he need only open the door a crack because
'longus amor tales corpus tenuauit in usus.'

733–4. **nec turpe putaris / palliolum nitidis inposuisse comis** : The
*palliolum* was a hood worn by invalids; Quintilian (xi. 3. 144)
decrees that for an orator 'palliolum . . . sola excusare potest
ualetudo.'

734. **nitidis . . . comis** : Ointment on the hair proclaimed a cheerful
party-goer (e.g. Horace, *Odes* i. iv. 9 'nunc decet aut uiridi
nitidum caput impedire myrto'), so revealing the illness as
something of a sham.

735. **uigilatae . . . noctes** : cf. *Amores* i. 2. 3 'et uacuus somno
noctem, quam longa, peregi', Propertius i. 1. 33, Tibullus iii. 4.
19–20, and the well-known figure in which all the world is asleep
but for the miserable lover (Ap. Rh. iii. 744 ff., Theocritus 2.
38 ff., *Aeneid* iv. 522 ff. etc.).

737–8. *You should be instantly recognizable as a lover.* For the motif
of an onlooker deducing from the appropriate symptoms that a
man is in love cf. Callimachus, *ep.* 43, Asclepiades, *Anth. Pal.* xii.
135 (= 18 Gow–Page), Horace, *Epodes* 11. 8 ff. 'conuiuiorum et
paenitet / in quis amantem languor et silentium / arguit et
latere petitus imo spiritus'.

738. **amas** : 'You must be in love.'

739–54. *Although it is shameful to admit, you cannot safely praise
your love to a friend, lest he supplant you.* The idea of a friend
trying to steal the poet's love occurs frequently (e.g. Catullus
77, Propertius ii. 34A); that the poet should lose her through
singing her praises is ingeniously taken up in *Amores* iii. 12. 7 ff.:

> fallimur, an nostris innotuit illa libellis?
> sic erit: ingenio prostitit illa meo.
> et merito: quid enim formae praeconia feci?
> uendibilis culpa facta puella mea est.

**739. conquerar an moneam . . . ? :** Kenney (in *Ovidiana*, p. 204 n. 4) points out that *conquestio* was a technical term in rhetoric (e.g. Cicero, *de Inventione* i. 106) and concludes that Ovid must mean 'Shall I indulge in rhetorical fireworks, or shall I get on with the work in hand, that of warning my readers?'

**mixtum fas omne nefasque :** cf. Virgil, *Georgics* i. 505 'quippe ubi fas uersum atque nefas', Seneca, *de Ira* ii. 9. 2 'undique uelut signo dato ad fas nefasque miscendum coorti sunt.'

**740. nomen amicitia est, nomen inane fides :** Mournful reflections on the fragility of friendship were commonplace (see Otto, *Sprichwörter*, s.v. Amicus 6 and 7); for the association with 'nomen' cf. Publilius Syrus 42 'amicum an nomen habeas, aperit calamitas', from Euripides, *Orestes* 454–5.

**nomen:** 'nothing but a word' cf. Horace, *Epist.* i. 6. 31 'uirtutem uerba putas', i. 17. 41 'aut uirtus nomen inane est'.

**743 ff.** As noted earlier, Kenney has suggested that the misplaced lines 585–8 could find a home after 742 (with 'tuta' emended to 'trita' in both 585 and 586). On balance I think that 'nomen amicitia est' (740) would be well picked up by 'per amici . . . nomen' (585).

**743–6.** A counter-argument by the imaginary objector: *true friends will not behave in so shocking a manner*. The three pairs mentioned (Patroclus and Achilles, Pirithous and Theseus, Pylades and Orestes) were proverbial for loyalty and affection (e.g. they are all mentioned together in Bion fr. 12 Gow).

**743.** Patroclus (Actorides from his grandfather Actor) did not try to interfere with Briseis, the young woman whom Achilles refused to surrender, thereby causing so many troubles to the Greeks.

**744.** The downfall of Theseus' wife Phaedra involved not Pirithous but her stepson Hippolytus (cf. 511).

**745–6.** Pylades had a pure affection for Orestes' wife Hermione, like that of Phoebus for the virgin goddess Athena, or of Castor and Pollux for their sister Helen.

**745.** Hermione, daughter of Menelaus and Helen, became the wife of Orestes after in some accounts being betrothed or even married to Neoptolemus.

**746.** 'And he [Pylades] was to her [Hermione] what the twins Castor and Pollux were to Helen.'

**geminus . . . Castor :** 'Castor and his twin'. We are clearly meant to think of both brothers, as in Horace, *Odes* iii. 29. 63–4 'tutum per Aegaeos tumultus / aura feret geminusque Pollux.'

**Tyndari :** Tyndareos was the husband of Leda and thus the putative father of Helen and the Dioscuri (who were normally held to be children of Jupiter). Concerning the use of the human patronymic for characters in this ambiguous position, see my note on *Met.* viii. 437.

**747–8.** Ovid's reply to the objector: *anyone who believes that must live in a world of fantasy, or expect that morals will be what they once were during the Golden Age.* Again we have the argument from the impossibility or ἀδύνατον (see on 271–2), but in a slightly unusual form. The commonest pattern is 'Sooner will a physical impossibility occur than such-and-such'; alternatively 'Since something quite incredible has happened, other equally extraordinary occurrences may follow' (e.g. Archilochus fr. 74, linked to an eclipse of the sun, Horace, *Odes* i. 29. 10 ff. (Iccius is selling his philosophical library), Ovid, *Tristia* i. 8. 1 ff. (the poet has been deceived by one whom he thought a friend)). Here the two propositions are on a level—if you can believe A, you will expect B.

**747. iacturas poma myricas :** Only an optimist would look for any kind of fruit from the *myrica* (tamarisk), as the shrub was notoriously barren (πανακαρπέα θάμνον Nicander, *Theriaca* 612, Pliny, *N.H.* xiii. 116, xxiv. 67). Though not strictly applicable here, one should also remember the commonplace of trees bearing unnatural fruits cf. Theocritus 1. 132 ff., Virgil, *Ecl.* 3. 89, 8. 52–4 'aurea durae / mala ferant quercus, narcisso floreat alnus, / pinguia corticibus sudent electra myricae.' It is significant that this motif, like 748, may be associated with the Golden Age, e.g. *Ecl.* 4. 29 'incultisque rubens pendebit sentibus uua'. Anyone who looks for loyalty between friends in a matter of love, says the poet, is demanding no less than the return of the ideal Golden Age.

The manuscripts offer a choice between 'iacturas' (better attested) and 'laturas'. We may concede to Goold (*Harvard Studies* 69 (1965), 67) that 'laturas' is the expected word; the question is whether Ovid may not for once have wished to surprise us. Why should not trees cast their fruit as well as bear it? Gronovius and Heinsius quoted Frontinus (*de Controversiis*, p. 10 ed. Thulin, *Corpus Agrimensorum Romanorum* I. i) 'quotiens (arbores) . . . fructum iactauerunt'; though Goold thinks little of this reference, it seems to me not altogether valueless. A Greek parallel would be [Moschus], *Lament for Bion* 32 δένδρεα καρπὸν ἔριψε. Perhaps one can also argue positively in favour of 'iacturas': a regular feature of the Golden Age is that everything came easily to man, who did not have to exert himself in any way. So here the tamarisk does not merely grow fruit but drops it into people's lap as well (cf. *Met.* i. 106 'et quae deciderant patula Iouis arbore glandes'—they do not even have to shake the tree). Note also comic parodies of the Golden Age in Athenaeus iv. 267e ff., particularly Pherecrates fr. 130 Edmonds ('deciduous bushes drop [φυλλοροήσει] fricasseed thrushes, and succulent gobbets of squid').

**748. e medio flumine mella petat :** cf. Virgil, *Ecl.* 3. 89 (among ἀδύνατα turned into a prayer for another's happiness and prosperity) 'mella fluant illi', inspired by Theocritus 5. 124–7. During the Golden Age such desirable liquids flowed freely for all (e.g. *Met.* i. 111 'flumina iam lactis, iam flumina nectaris ibant' with Bömer's note).

**751–2.** The mournful tone recalls Theognis (and Pseudo-Theognis) who is for ever bewailing the fragility of friendship and the fact that false friends can be more dangerous than open enemies (e.g. *Theognidea* 1219–20 West ἐχθρὸν μὲν χαλεπὸν καὶ δυσμενῆ ἐξαπατῆσαι,/ Κύρνε· φίλον δὲ φίλῳ ῥᾴδιον ἐξαπατᾶν).

**753. cognatum fratremque caue carumque sodalem :** on the disruptive power of love cf. Propertius ii. 34. 5–6 'polluit ille deus cognatos, soluit amicos, / et bene concordes tristia ad arma uocat.' Just as 747–8 suggested the Golden Age, so here we should think of standard denunciations of moral decline thereafter. Often mentioned is disloyalty between close relatives and friends, e.g. *Met.* i. 144–5 'non hospes ab hospite tutus / non socer a genero, fratrum quoque gratia rara est.' The *topos* (fully illustrated by Bömer ad loc.) goes back to Hesiod; for sexual jealousy resulting cf. Catullus 64. 401–2.

**755–70.** *A final word: the nature of women is infinitely varied, and you must be infinitely resourceful in catching the one of your choice.*

**755. finiturus eram :** Similar touches suggesting infirmity of purpose are iii. 193 'quam paene admonui', 612 'praeteriturus eram'. One might compare Virgil, *Georgics* iv. 116 ff., but closer is the opening of Manilius v 'hic alius finisset iter, signisque relatis . . . / . . . non ultra struxisset opus.'

**755–6. sed sunt diuersa puellis / pectora :** So didactic poems on hunting or fishing will stress the great variety of the prey, e.g. Oppian, *Hal.* i. 93–4 ἰχθύσι μὲν γενεή τε καὶ ἤθεα καὶ πόρος ἅλμης / κέκριται, οὐδέ τι πᾶσι νομαὶ νεπόδεσσιν ὁμοῖαι.

**756. excipe :** 'catch', often used as a hunting term (Horace, *Odes* iii. 12. 12, Propertius ii. 19. 24).

**757–8. nec tellus eadem parit omnia : uitibus illa / conuenit, haec oleis ; hic bene farra uirent :** switching our thoughts to Virgil, *Georgics* ii. 109 'nec uero terrae ferre omnes omnia possunt' and i. 54 'hic segetes, illic ueniunt felicius uuae' (quoted by Kenney in *Ovidiana*, p. 207).

**759. pectoribus mores tot sunt, quot in ore figurae :** There are as many varieties of character as of facial looks. Bentley's correction 'ore' for 'orbe' restores point and balance to the comparison (for 'in ore figurae' Kenney cites Terence, *Eunuchus* 317 'noua figura oris', Cicero, *de Or.* i. 114 'figura totius oris et corporis').

**761–2.** On the transformations of Proteus cf. *Odyssey* iv. 456 ff. (where the possibilities include a snake and a leopard), Virgil,

*Georgics* iv. 407 ff. (also a tiger and fire), Ovid, *Met.* viii. 731 ff. (also a stone and a bull).

**761. tenuabit :** 'He (the lover) will, like Proteus, make himself melt into insubstantial water (i.e. show extreme versatility).' The correction 'tenuabit' for 'tenuauit' receives support, if that were necessary, from λεπτυνεῖ in a Byzantine translation (*Ovidiana Graeca, ed.* Easterling and Kenney, *Proc. Cam. Phil. Soc.* Suppl. 1 (1965), p. 25).

**762. nunc leŏ :** the only example of the nominative in elegy (and indeed the whole of Ovid) which suggests that the poets felt an inhibition about the quantity. Virgil will happily write leō.

**763–4.** Compare Oppian, *Hal.* iii. 72–3 τέτραχα δ' εἰναλίης θήρης νόμον ἐφράσσαντο / ἰχθυβόλοι (his four methods are hook, net, basket-trap, and trident).

**763. iaculo :** not a harpoon (the ancient fish-spear, a trident, was thrust rather than thrown) but a casting-net; *iaculum* is neuter of the adjective with 'rete' understood. In this couplet Ovid distinguishes between casting-nets and drag-nets (*trahunt,* 764), respectively ἀμφίβληστρα and γρῖφοι (Oppian, *Hal.* iii. 80, see Mair's Introduction, pp. xl–xliii).

**764. caua :** 'bulging'. The epithet conveys the idea of enclosing and enfolding (cf. *Aeneid* ii. 360 'nox atra caua circumuolat umbra').

**766. cerua . . . anus :** famed for both longevity (e.g. Juvenal 14. 251 'longa et ceruina senectus') and timorousness. The same thought may be applied to other animals (see Otto, s.v. Lupus 7). The variant 'curua . . . anus' drew the scorn of Heinsius: 'Ridicule profecto. Causae scilicet multum est cur anus iam curuata prae senio insidias amatorum metuat.'

**767–70.** One of the few occasions when a genuine kindness (which I can believe Ovid to have possessed as a person) seems to break through the glittering surface of the *Ars.*

**771–2. Pars superat coepti, pars est exhausta, laboris : / hic teneat nostras ancora iacta rates :** A breathing-point marking the end of book i and half the projected task (*pars . . . pars*); this couplet derives from the original scheme of the work in only two books (see Introduction, p. xii), and Ovid did not trouble to obliterate it when adding book iii. At exactly the corresponding place in Virgil's *Georgics* (ii. 541–2) we read 'sed nos immensum spatiis confecimus aequor, / et iam tempus equum fumantia soluere colla'—Ovid has changed the chariot-image to that of a ship (for these two, see on 39–40). Compare also *Georgics* iii. 286 'hoc satis armentis. superat pars altera curae.'

# APPENDIX I

## The Chronology of Ovid's Earlier Works and the *Ars*

THE account given in my Introduction (pp. xi–xii) of Ovid's poetic career up to the writing of the *Ars* inevitably contains an element of speculation. I believe it to be the most plausible, but some scholars have taken different views. Controversy centres around *Amores* ii. 18, involving the *Amores*, *Heroides*, the lost tragedy *Medea*, and the *Ars Amatoria*. Alan Cameron, in an article much of which I agree with (*CQ* N.S. 18 (1968), 320–33), is the latest to deny that the poem was written for the second edition of the *Amores*, or that line 19 ('quod licet, aut *artes* teneri profitemur *Amoris*') refers to the *Ars Amatoria*.

Cameron (p. 332) offers a number of arguments which, if valid, would more or less compel assent to his position:

(i) 'To accept this (sc. that *Am.* ii. 18. 19 refers to the *Ars*) would entail accepting that the second edition of the *Amores* appeared after *Ars* i–ii' (on p. 331 Cameron mentions the date of *c.* A.D. 2, which in any case is two or three years later than necessary). But why? 'Artes . . . profitemur Amoris' naturally means 'I am working on an *Ars Amatoria*', not 'I have completed and published the poem.' The *Ars* could still be in quite a rudimentary condition; a date of around 6 B.C. (which Cameron on p. 333 implies for the second edition of the *Amores*) seems perfectly appropriate.

(ii) '*Amores* ii. 18. 13–14 clearly implies that Ovid had *not* yet written a tragedy.' The couplet runs 'sceptra tamen sumpsi curaque tragoedia nostra / creuit, et huic operi quamlibet aptus eram' (thereafter Cupid laughs and recalls the poet to lighter themes). Presumably Cameron would infer that the tragedy was abandoned half-complete, which may be too literal an interpretation of the motif. But I am inclined to draw the opposite conclusion: Ovid *has* finished the *Medea*, yet, in spite of its favourable reception ('et huic operi quamlibet aptus eram') he is still wedded to love-poetry and has not become a regular tragedian. Some older scholars (rightly, I think) gave a capital to 'Tragoedia', 'and Tragedy was increased through my efforts.' This personification appears in *Amores* iii. 1, and I see here Ovid's response to her demand 'nunc habeam per te Romana Tragoedia nomen'

(iii. 1. 29). Note that 'creuit' would then bear a multiplicity of meanings in true Ovidian style: (a) 'was increased' (the corpus of tragedy had one play added to it), (b) 'gained in esteem', (c) 'swelled with pride', (d) 'grew larger'—perhaps one should think of deities who suddenly expand (e.g. Demeter in Callimachus, *hymn* 6 or Fama in *Aeneid* iv), also of figures like Horace, *Odes* i. 1. 35–6 'quodsi me lyricis uatibus inseres / sublimi feriam sidera uertice.'

(iii) '*Amores* iii. 1 and iii. 15 clearly represent Ovid as much nearer completing his *Medea* than ii. 18.' For ii. 18 see above. As to iii. 1 and iii. 15, they both express a wish to write tragedy in the future, but (with the conceivable though very doubtful exception of iii. 1. 63–4) give no hint that he has already started to do so.

In conclusion, I do believe that *Amores* ii. 18. 19 describes the *Ars Amatoria*; both the near approximation to the title (artes . . . Amoris) and the stress on a sustained teaching role (profitemur) make this the natural inference. So *Amores* ii. 18 was probably added for the second edition, while iii. 1 and iii. 15 should be placed among the last of the first edition (with iii. 15 a likely 'seal' to the five-book collection).

# APPENDIX II

## 'Me Venus artificem tenero praefecit Amori' (7): Bion fr. 10 Gow

Ἁ μεγάλα μοι Κύπρις ἔθ' ὑπνώοντι παρέστα
νηπίαχον τὸν Ἔρωτα καλᾶς ἐκ χειρὸς ἄγοισα
ἐς χθόνα νευστάζοντα, τόσον δέ μοι ἔφρασε μῦθον·
'μέλπειν μοι, φίλε βοῦτα, λαβὼν τὸν Ἔρωτα δίδασκε'.
ὣς λέγε· χἀ μὲν ἀπῆλθεν, ἐγὼ δ' ὅσα βουκολίασδον,
νήπιος ὣς ἐθέλοντα μαθεῖν, τὸν Ἔρωτα δίδασκον,
ὡς εὗρεν πλαγίαυλον ὁ Πάν, ὡς αὐλὸν Ἀθάνα,
ὡς χέλυν Ἑρμάων, κίθαριν ὡς ἁδὺς Ἀπόλλων.
ταῦτά νιν ἐξεδίδασκον· ὁ δ' οὐκ ἐμπάζετο μύθων,
ἀλλά μοι αὐτὸς ἄειδεν ἐρωτύλα, καί με δίδασκε
θνατῶν ἀθανάτων τε πόθως καὶ ματέρος ἔργα.
κἠγὼν ἐκλαθόμαν μὲν ὅσων τὸν Ἔρωτα δίδασκον,
ὅσσα δ' Ἔρως με δίδαξεν ἐρωτύλα πάντα διδάχθην.

I slept, when Venus enter'd: to my bed
A Cupid in her beauteous hand she led,
A bashful-seeming boy, and thus she said:
'Shepherd, receive my little one! I bring
An untaught love, whom thou must teach to sing.'
She said, and left him. I suspecting nought
Many a sweet strain my subtle pupil taught,
How reed to reed Pan first with osier bound,
How Pallas form'd the pipe of softest sound,
How Hermes gave the lute, and how the quire
Of Phoebus owe to Phoebus' self the lyre.
Such were my themes; my themes nought heeded he,
But ditties sang of am'rous sort to me,
The pangs that mortals and immortals prove
From Venus' influence, and the darts of love.
Thus was the teacher by the pupil taught;
His lessons I retain'd, and mine forgot.

WILLIAM COWPER

# APPENDIX III

## Another *Propempticon* for Gaius: Antipater of Thessalonica, *Anth. Pal.* ix. 297 = Antipater no. 47 Gow–Page (*The Garland of Philip*)

Στέλλευ ἐπ' Εὐφρήτην, Ζηνὸς τέκος· εἰς σὲ γὰρ ἤδη
ἠῷοι Πάρθων αὐτομολοῦσι πόδες.
στέλλευ, ἄναξ· δήεις δὲ φόβῳ κεχαλασμένα τόξα,
Καῖσαρ· πατρῴων δ' ἄρξαι ἀπ' ἐντολέων·
'Ρώμην δ', 'Ωκεανῷ περιτέρμονα πάντοθεν, αὐτὸς
πρῶτος ἀνερχομένῳ σφράγισαι ἠελίῳ.

'Be on your way to the Euphrates, son of Zeus; to you already the Parthians in the East are deserting apace. Be on your way, my prince; you shall find their bows unstrung through terror, Caesar. Rule in accord with your father's precepts, and be yourself the first to certify to the rising sun that Rome is bounded by the ocean on all sides.'

I give the translation of Gow–Page, who recognize that the exact interpretation of the last three lines can be disputed. Antipater probably lived in Rome at this time, enjoying the patronage of L. Calpurnius Piso Frugi (cos. 15 B.C.). Since we can trace other links between Antipater and Ovid (both address the Thracian prince Cotys, and write dawn-poems resembling each other), it seems quite likely that the two poets were personally acquainted.

For the historical background see my introductory note to 177–228. Some parallels with Ovid are clear: the prophecy that Gaius will extend Roman power to the extreme East (Antipater 6, cf. Ovid 178 'nunc, Oriens ultime, noster eris') and the close dependence of Gaius on his adoptive father (Antipater 4, Ovid 191 'auspiciis annisque patris, puer, arma mouebis'). A problem arises from lines 1–2, which Gow–Page surely misinterpret in their commentary. These words must refer not to any willingness by the Parthian king Phraataces to make concessions (in fact he was quite intransigent at first), but rather to disaffection among his people, mentioned also by Dio (lv. 10ᵃ. 4). The Parthians who deserted to Gaius were presumably nobles who supported one of the hostage princes in Rome against Phraataces and crossed over to the Roman side to join them.

# APPENDIX IV

## Busiris and Phalaris in Callimachus' *Aetia*

J U S T enough remains of the fragments of the *Aetia* to show that in lines 647–56 Ovid imitated Callimachus closely[1]. One hexameter referring to Busiris has come down to us, probably the opening one (fr. 44):

> Αἴγυπτος προπάροιθεν ἐπ' ἐννέα κάρφετο ποίας

'Egypt previously was parched for nine summers.'

This is translated almost word for word by Ovid in 647–8. A stray pentameter (fr. 45) indicates that Callimachus had the stories in the same order:

> τὴν κείνου Φάλαρις πρῆξιν ἀπεπλάσατο

'Phalaris copied his (i.e. Busiris') deed.'

It is tempting (though not certainly right) to place immediately after fr. 45 the couplet fr. 46 of which Perillus is the subject:

> πρῶτος ἐπεὶ τὸν ταῦρον ἐκαίνισεν, ὃς τὸν ὄλεθρον
> εὗρε τὸν ἐν χαλκῷ καὶ πυρὶ γιγνόμενον

'since the first man to try out the bull was he who invented the death which comes from fire and bronze'.

Note that Ovid's 'imbuit' (654) corresponds exactly to ἐκαίνισεν in Callimachus.

Some scholars have attempted to recover another fragment on Phalaris from an anonymous proverb in the Suda: τοῦτο ποήσας / τῶν ἀδίκων ἔργων ἐν τὸ δικαιότατον ('doing thereby the one of his unjust deeds which was supremely just'). This could provide a sort of link with Ovid 655 'iustus uterque fuit', but Pfeiffer was rightly sceptical (see the note to fr. 46 in his Addenda, vol. I, p. 500) while admitting that Callimachus might have used the proverb in some other form.

[1] Since this Appendix was written, I gather that a new papyrus has come to light, linking up with fr. 46— a reminder that the process of rediscovery continues.

# APPENDIX V

## [Bion], Epithalamion of Achilles and Deidamia, lines 10–30

ἅρπασε τὰν ῾Ελέναν πόθ᾽ ὁ βωκόλος, ἆγε δ᾽ ἐς ῎Ιδαν,      10
Οἰνώνῃ κακὸν ἄλγος. ἐχώσατο δ᾽ ἁ Λακεδαίμων
πάντα δὲ λαὸν ἄγειρεν Ἀχαϊκόν, οὐδέ τις ῞Ελλην,
οὔτε Μυκηναίων οὔτ᾽ ῎Ηλιδος οὔτε Λακώνων
μεῖνεν ἑὸν κατὰ δῶμα φυγὼν δύστανον Ἄρηα.
λάνθανε δ᾽ ἐν κώραις Λυκομηδίσι μοῦνος Ἀχιλλεύς,      15
εἴρια δ᾽ ἀνθ᾽ ὅπλων ἐδιδάσκετο, καὶ χερὶ λευκᾷ
παρθενικὸν κόρον εἶχεν, ἐφαίνετο δ᾽ ἠύτε κώρα·
καὶ γὰρ ἴσον τήναις θηλύνετο, καὶ τόσον ἄνθος
χιονέαις πόρφυρε παρηίσι, καὶ τὸ βάδισμα
παρθενικῆς ἐβάδιζε, κόμας δ᾽ ἐπύκαζε καλύπτρῃ.      20
θυμὸν δ᾽ ἀνέρος εἶχε καὶ ἀνέρος εἶχεν ἔρωτα·
ἐξ ἀοῦς δ᾽ ἐπὶ νύκτα παρίζετο Δηιδαμείᾳ,
καὶ ποτὲ μὲν τήνας ἐφίλει χέρα, πολλάκι δ᾽ αὐτᾶς
στάμονα καλὸν ἄειρε τὰ δαίδαλα δ᾽ ἄτρι᾽ ἐπήνει·
ἤσθιε δ᾽ οὐκ ἄλλᾳ σὺν ὁμάλικι, πάντα δ᾽ ἐποίει      25
σπεύδων κοινὸν ἐς ὕπνον, ἔλεξέ νυ καὶ λόγον αὐτᾷ·
῾ἄλλαι μὲν κνώσσουσι σὺν ἀλλήλαισιν ἀδελφαί,
αὐτὰρ ἐγὼ μούνα, μούνα δὲ σύ, νύμφα, καθεύδεις.
αἱ δύο παρθενικαὶ συνομάλικες, αἱ δύο καλαί,
ἀλλὰ μόναι κατὰ λέκτρα καθεύδομες . . .᾽      30

'Once the herdsman made off with Helen and brought her to Ida, a bitter pain for Oenone. Sparta was enraged, and gathered together all the Achaean people; no Greek, whether from Mycenae, Elis, or Laconia, stayed at home to avoid the miseries of war. Only Achilles hid himself away among the daughters of Lycomedes, and learned of wool rather than weapons; in his pale hand he held a maiden's broom, and his appearance was that of a girl. For he was as soft as they; there was no less a bloom on his snow-white cheeks when he blushed, he walked like a girl and confined his hair with a veil. But he had the spirit and the passion of a male. From morning till night he sat by Deidamia. Sometimes he would kiss her hand, and often he lifted up her warp, and praised the intricate work; with no other companion did he eat, and strove in every way to spend the night with her. And he reasoned with her as well: "The other sisters sleep one with another, but I sleep alone, and so do you, maiden—both of us virgins and friends, both fair, and yet we sleep alone in our beds . . ." '

# APPENDIX VI

## Select Bibliography

### (1) EDITIONS

BORNECQUE, H., *Ars Amatoria*, with brief notes (Budé), Paris, 1939.

BRANDT, P., *Ars Amatoria*, with commentary, Leipzig, 1902.

BURMAN, P., *Opera*, with notes of N. Heinsius and others, vol. I, Amsterdam, 1727.

EHWALD, R., *Opera*, vol. I, Leipzig, 1888.

GRIGGS, M. J., *Ars Amatoria*, selections with notes, London, 1971.

KENNEY, E. J., *Ars Amatoria* and other love poems, Oxford Classical Texts, 1961, reprinted from corrected sheets, 1965.

LENZ, F. W., *Ars Amatoria*, with brief notes, Turin, 1969 (Corpus Scriptorum Latinorum Paravianum).

—— *Ars Amatoria* with fuller commentary, Berlin, 1969.

MOZLEY, J. H., *Ars Amatoria* etc. (Loeb), 1929.

VARIORUM, *Opera*, vol. I, with notes of Bentley and others, Oxford, 1826.

### (2) OTHER BOOKS

BALSDON, J. P. V. D., *Life and Leisure in Ancient Rome*, London, 1969.

BEARE, W., *The Roman Stage*, 3rd ed., London, 1968.

BINNS, J. W. (ed.), *Ovid*, London, 1973.

DEFERRARI, R. J., BARRY, M. I., and McGUIRE, M. R. P., *A Concordance of Ovid*, Washington, 1939.

DÖPP, S., *Virgilischer Einfluß im Werk Ovids*, Munich, 1969.

FRÄNKEL, H., *Ovid, a Poet between Two Worlds*, Berkeley, Cal., 1945.

HERESCU, N. I. (ed.), *Ovidiana*, Paris, 1958.

LENZ, F. W., *Opuscula Selecta* (many Ovidian articles), Amsterdam, 1972.

LILJA, S., *The Roman Elegists' Attitude to Women*, Helsinki, 1965.

MUNARI, F., *Il Codice Hamilton 471 di Ovidio*, Rome, 1965.

NASH, E., *Pictorial Dictionary of Ancient Rome*, 2 vols., London, 1961–2.

OTTO, A., *Die Sprichwörter der Römer*, Leipzig, 1890.

PICHON, R., *De Sermone Amatorio apud Latinos Elegiarum Scriptores*, Paris, 1902.

PLATNAUER, M., *Latin Elegiac Verse*, Cambridge, 1951.

PLATNER, S. B., and ASHBY, T., *A Topographical Dictionary of Ancient Rome*, Oxford, 1929.

THIBAULT, J. C., *The Mystery of Ovid's Exile*, Berkeley, Cal., 1964.

TURNER, P., Ovid, *The Technique of Love and Remedies for Love* (prose translations), London, 1968.

WILKINSON, L. P., *Ovid Recalled*, Cambridge, 1955.

WILSON, Lillian M., *The Clothing of the Ancient Romans*, Baltimore, 1938.


(3) ARTICLES, ETC.

BRUNT, P. A., 'Pay and Superannuation in the Roman Army', *BSR* 18 (1950), 50–71.

—— review of Meyer, 'Die Außenpolitik des Augustus und die Augusteische Dichtung', *JRS* 53 (1963), 170–6.

CAMERON, Alan, 'The First Edition of Ovid's *Amores*', *CQ* N.S. 18 (1968), 320–33.

GALINSKY, Karl, 'The Triumph Theme in the Augustan Elegy', *Wiener Studien* N.S. 3 (1969), 75–107.

GARIÉPY, R. J., Jnr., 'Recent Scholarship on Ovid (1958–68)', *CW* 64. 2 (Oct. 1970), 37–56.

GOOLD, G. P., 'Amatoria Critica', *HSCP* 69 (1965), 1–107.

HOLLIS, A. S., '*Ars Amatoria* and *Remedia Amoris*', in *Ovid*, ed. Binns (see section 2 above), pp. 84–115.

KENNEY, E. J., Unpublished dissertation on text of the *Ars* (partly reproduced in later published notes).

—— 'Ovid, *Ars Amatoria* i. 147', *CR* N.S. 3 (1953), 7–10.

—— 'Nequitiae Poeta', in *Ovidiana* (see section 2 above, Herescu), pp. 201–9.

—— 'Notes on Ovid: II', *CQ* N.S. 9 (1959), 240–60.

—— 'The Manuscript Tradition of Ovid's *Amores*, *Ars Amatoria*, and *Remedia Amoris*', *CQ* N.S. 12 (1962), 1–31.

—— 'Ovid and the Law', *YCS* 21 (1969), 243–63.

LA PIANA, G., 'Foreign Groups in Rome', *Harvard Theological Review*, 20 (1927), 183–403.

LEACH, Eleanor, 'Georgic Imagery in the *Ars Amatoria*', *TAPA* 95 (1964), 142–54.

OTIS, B., 'Ovid and the Augustans', *TAPA* 69 (1938), 188–229.

REYNOLDS, R. W., 'The Adultery Mime', *CQ* 40 (1946), 77–84.

RUDD, Niall, 'Ovid and the Augustan Myth', in *Lines of Enquiry* (Cambridge, 1976), 1–31.

SCOTT, K., 'Emperor Worship in Ovid', *TAPA* 61 (1930), 43–69.

SUERBAUM, W., 'Ovid über seine Inspiration', *Hermes* 93 (1965), 491–6.

SYME, R. 'The Crisis of 2 B.C.', *Bayerische Akad. der Wissenschaften, phil.-hist. KL. S-B.* 1974, 7.

THOMAS, Elizabeth, 'Ovid at the Races', in 'Hommages à Marcel Renard', ed. J. Bibauw, vol. I (Collections Latomus 101 (1969)), pp. 710–24.

TRÄNKLE, H., 'Textkritische und exegetische Bemerkungen zu Ovids *Ars Amatoria*', *Hermes* 100 (1972), 387–408.

WARDMAN, A. E., 'The Rape of the Sabines', *CQ* N.S. 15 (1965), 101–3.

# INDEX OF ANCIENT AUTHORS AND PASSAGES CITED

Figures after the colon denote page numbers. A few less interesting references from an Ovidian viewpoint have been omitted

# GENERAL INDEX